"Chronic pain is like a weed that can take over the landscape of your life if you let it. Yet, it doesn't have to be this way. This remarkable and beautifully written book offers a fresh approach to a life defined by chronic pain and its management. Readers will learn how to get out of a life consumed with pain and pain management and back into a life where pain takes a backseat. This book, filled with many well-crafted examples and exercises, will teach you skills that will help you learn to be with your pain and live a vital life. You will learn how to bring compassion and acceptance to your pain and hurt while engaging in actions that you care deeply about. This book is a vital resource for those suffering from chronic pain, their loved ones, and professionals who work to help people who are stuck and suffering in a cycle of pain and misery."

—*John P. Forsyth, Ph.D., associate professor of psychology and faculty director of the Anxiety Disorders Research Program, State University of New York at Albany*

"This easy-to-read workbook was written for people who are exhausted and frustrated by their unsuccessful efforts to overcome pain. It's a life-affirming guide that shows readers a way to free themselves from the shackles of all those tedious pain management and control programs and how to get back into the life they have put on hold—a life that is devoted to pursuing the things that really matter to them. Dahl and Lundgren teach readers in clear practical steps how to get back into the driver's seat of their "life-bus" by accepting pain, avoiding getting bogged down by painful thinking, and starting to move in a direction that is determined by what they truly value."

—*Georg H. Eifert, Ph.D., professor and chair of psychology at Chapman University and author of* Acceptance and Commitment Therapy for Anxiety Disorders, ACT on Life Not on Anger, *and* The Anorexia Workbook

Living Beyond Your Pain

Using Acceptance & Commitment
Therapy to Ease Chronic Pain

JOANNE DAHL, PH.D. & TOBIAS LUNDGREN, MS

New Harbinger Publications, Inc.

Distributed in Canada by Raincoast Books.

Copyright © 2006 by JoAnne Dahl and Tobias Lundgren
New Harbinger Publications, Inc.
5674 Shattuck Avenue
Oakland, CA 94609
www.newharbinger.com

Cover design by Amy Shoup; Acquired by Melissa Kirk;
Edited by Jasmine Star; Text design by Tracy Marie Carlson

Library of Congress Cataloging-in-Publication Data

Dahl, JoAnne, 1951-
   Living beyond your pain : using acceptance and commitment therapy to ease chronic pain / JoAnne Dahl and Tobias Lundgren.
       p. cm.
   ISBN-13: 978-1-57224-409-2
   ISBN-10: 1-57224-409-7
   1. Chronic pain—Treatment. 2. Acceptance and commitment therapy. I. Lundgren, Tobias. II. Title.
   RB127.D35 2006
   616'.0472—dc22

                                        2006002532

Printed in the United States of America

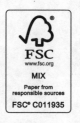
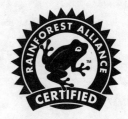

19 18 17

15 14 13 12 11 10

To my mother, Caroline, who instilled in me the courage to show my light. Although you have been gone for nearly forty years, your loving presence is always with me.

—J.A.D.

I dedicate this book to the spirit of the ocean, the vitality of the Liverpool Football Club, and my love for my brothers.

—T.L.L.

Contents

Foreword

THE QUESTION LIFE IS ASKING

Life is asking you a question, and it requires a yes or a no answer. The question has been there a long time, but it probably took a while to begin to hear it. Very likely you have now sensed that the question is there, and that's probably part of why you have picked up this book. If the answer to this question is yes, this is a book worth reading. If the answer is no, it's not. Only you can give the answer. I will tell you the question at the end of this foreword, and you will be able to decide for yourself if this book is for you.

There are two kinds of pain. One kind you feel when it comes out of the background and presents itself. The second kind you feel when something is *not* there.

Initially, chronic pain seems to be more a matter of the first kind. Uninvited, unwanted, bodily sensations seem to be saying that something is wrong; something can and must be fixed. The logical, reasonable, sensible thing to do is to find out what that something is—and get it fixed.

Meanwhile, life itself must seemingly be put on hold. Compromises need to be made while a fight against pain is fought and won. But the weeks turn into months, and the months turn into years. The war rages on; the distress and sense of desperation grows. The life compromises become deeper, and they broaden into more and more areas.

The book you have in your hand presents a profound alternative to continuing to fight that war. It raises the realistic possibility that it is time to start living again. Really living. Now.

How is that possible if pain will not leave? What else can be done when the logical, reasonable, sensible things have all failed to provide an answer? This book shows you the alternative and why it might work. It walks you through the skills you will need to transform your life.

This volume reviews the sad evidence that trying to reduce pain, per se, is not a powerful way to approach chronic pain. Then it skillfully and carefully puts on the table the Acceptance and Commitment Therapy model instead ("ACT," said as a single word, not as initials; Hayes & Smith, 2005, Hayes, Strosahl, & Wilson 1999). The ACT model refocuses your life. In the service of what you truly value, it teaches you to contact the present moment more fully as a conscious human being, feeling what you feel and thinking what you think, and to move in the direction of a life worth living. Now.

What justifies giving it a chance is the second kind of pain: the kind that comes when something is not there. Struggles with chronic pain can disconnect you from your life—from your family, spouse, children, friends, work, and recreation. This can be the greatest pain of all. It is that unavoidable fact that makes sense of the unusual skills you will learn from this excellent presentation of the ACT model by experts who have pioneered its application in the field of chronic pain (Dahl, Wilson, Luciano & Hayes 2005).

And here we arrive at the question life is asking. Given all that you've suffered and all that putting your life on hold has cost you, are you ready for something new—truly new? Have you suffered enough? If the answer is yes, this book is for you. If the answer is no, it is not.

Even though what is in this book may be new to you, it's not untested. It is based on an extensive program of psychological science, both basic (Hayes, Barnes-Holmes, & Roche 2001) and applied (Hayes, Luoma, Bond, Masuda, & Lillis 2006). It has been tested with pain, in the laboratory (Hayes et al. 1999), in preventative, work-based programs (Dahl, Wilson, & Nilsson 2004), and in the clinic (McCracken, Vowles, & Eccleston 2005). We know these methods can be helpful.

You are about to enter into new territory. It is both exciting and scary to step into the unknown, but as a wit once said, if you always do what you've always done, you will always get what you've always gotten. You have answered yes to the key question. Enough is enough. It is time to take a new path.

Out of caring for your own suffering, turn the page and begin.

—Steven C. Hayes
University of Nevada

REFERENCES

Dahl, J., K. G. Wilson, C. Luciano, & S. C. Hayes. 2005. *Acceptance and Commitment Therapy for Chronic Pain.* Reno, NV: Context Press.

Dahl, J., K. G. Wilson, & A. Nilsson. 2004. Acceptance and Commitment Therapy and the treatment of persons at risk for long-term disability resulting from stress and pain symptoms: A preliminary randomized trial. *Behavior Therapy* 35:785-802.

Hayes, S. C., D. Barnes-Holmes, & B. Roche, eds. 2001. *Relational Frame Theory: A Post-Skinnerian Account of Human Language and Cognition.* New York: Plenum Press.

Hayes, S. C., R. Bissett, Z. Korn, R. D. Zettle, I. Rosenfarb, L. Cooper, & A. Grundt. 1999. The impact of acceptance versus control rationales on pain tolerance. *The Psychological Record* 49:33-47.

Hayes, S. C., J. Luoma, F. Bond, A. Masuda, and J. Lillis. 2006. Acceptance and Commitment Therapy: Model, processes, and outcomes. *Behaviour Research and Therapy* 44:1-25.

Hayes, S. C. & S. Smith. 2005. *Get Out of Your Mind and into Your Life: The new Acceptance and Commitment Therapy.* Oakland, CA: New Harbinger.

Hayes, S. C., K. Strosahl, & K. G. Wilson. 1999. *Acceptance and Commitment Therapy: An Experiential Approach to Behavior Change.* New York: Guilford Press.

McCracken, L. M, K. E. Vowles, & C. Eccleston. 2005. Acceptance-based treatment for persons with complex, long-standing chronic pain: A preliminary analysis of treatment outcome in comparison to a waiting phase. *Behaviour Research and Therapy* 43:1335-1346.

Introduction

If you've picked up this book, you probably suffer from chronic pain. As such, you have faced some of the most terrible and difficult circumstances a person can face. You've had to cope with the physical and psychological symptoms of an ongoing ache that never seems to let up or end. You've suffered physically, and you've suffered psychologically. And if your pain has been going on for some time, as we expect it has, you may have watched it eat away at your life. As your pain has gotten bigger and bigger, your life has gotten smaller and smaller. You used to live a life that you loved. Now your life is devoted to trying to keep the pain at bay. In fact, you may not even be able to tell who's making the decisions about your life at this point—you or your pain.

You may feel as though you're sinking in quicksand and that slowly, over time, the pain has sucked you under. You can hardly move your arms or legs anymore, and you fear you may soon be completely engulfed by this terrible chronic condition. What's worse, it may seem as though every move you make to get out of pain just aggravates the situation. You struggle with the pain, and the more you struggle, the more it sucks you under. Perhaps you feel as though your suffering will never end.

If you know anything about quicksand, you might be starting to wonder whether your struggle with pain is what's sucking you under. When you're mired in actual quicksand, the more you struggle, the more inexorably it pulls you down. Each time you lift one foot, your other foot sinks more deeply into the quicksand.

In fact, there's only one way to extract yourself from the quicksand's pull. You have to work *with* the quicksand. You have to lie out on it spread-eagled and touch it with as much of the surface area of your body as you can; this allows it to support you rather than drag you under. You have to accept your predicament and get in touch with it on a very real and physical level. If you don't, the struggle will continue endlessly (Hayes, Strosahl, and Wilson 1999).

This is not another physical therapy book. We're not going to teach you ways to reduce your pain. We're not going to give you another new set of strategies that won't work. After all, you've probably tried just about everything that's out there: physical therapy, painkillers, and alternative therapies. How many books on bodywork have you read? How many of them have reduced your pain? We're betting that the answer is zero, otherwise you wouldn't have opened this book.

What we're going to suggest in this book is probably radically different than anything you've read or heard about until now. It has the potential to change your relationship with your pain enough that you can start to live your life in ways you may have thought would never be possible again. And you can begin to experience that transformation right away.

This book is founded on a premise that goes back to the quicksand metaphor we just introduced you to. Pain is very much like quicksand. The more you fight against it, the more of your life it takes away. The harder you struggle, the more it pulls you down. There's only one way out: You need to come into contact with your pain in order to be free from it. Since you can't get rid of your pain, you need to lie spread-eagled on it and touch it with every surface of your being. You need to realize that it may not go away. And you need to learn to live your life with this pain rather than letting it take your life away from you.

ACCEPTANCE AND COMMITMENT THERAPY FOR PAIN: VICTORY THROUGH SURRENDER

This book is built on the principles of acceptance and commitment therapy (ACT), a groundbreaking new psychological treatment approach developed by Steven Hayes and colleagues Kirk Strosahl and Kelly Wilson. This approach is built on a sound scientific foundation and has been used to treat people with chronic pain (Dahl, Wilson, and Nilsson 2004), as well as other chronic problems such as depression, substance abuse, eating disorders, and diabetes, with astonishing results (Zettle and Hayes 1986; Luciano et al. 2001; Heffner and Eifert 2004; Gregg 2004).

The ACT approach to pain involves two fundamental concepts. The first is that you must accept the aspects of your pain that you cannot change, including all of the difficult thoughts, feelings, and bodily sensations that come with it. The second is that this acceptance allows you to open a space where you can commit to acting in ways that make you feel vital and energized.

ACT is not about eliminating pain. In fact, you'll find out that one of the fundamental tenets of ACT is that pain can't be avoided. So while this book promises to help you with your pain problem, it won't help you escape pain. What it will help you do is learn to accept your pain for what it is and begin living the life you want to live starting today. Pain is only one part of the complete experience that is your life. ACT promises to change the way you relate to your pain so you can experience your life fully. Accepting your pain to live your life is what we call "victory by surrender."

THE AIM OF THIS WORKBOOK

This workbook aims to help you approach your predicament with chronic pain in a way that will get you out of the quicksand you're caught in and back into living the life you want to live. The ACT approach will teach you that much of what you think and feel and do in regard to your pain is like fighting to get out of quicksand. Resisting what you cannot control in regard to your pain, including your thoughts and feelings about it, will distance you from taking joy in life and living in accord with your values. Fighting pain is a losing battle, and it results in feelings of emptiness, alienation, and self-blame.

The key thought in the ACT approach to chronic pain is that you can accept your pain and live a valued life with it rather than allowing it to control you and minimize the vitality you feel every day. You do this by letting go of the control strategies you've been using to reduce pain, instead starting to live how you want to. ACT is about taking back the driver's seat in your life, steering where you most want to go, and inviting pain along as a valued passenger. This implies that there's nothing wrong with the pain experience itself, and indeed it's absolutely necessary for our survival. Pain is usually a message from the body to the brain that something is wrong and needs attention. The difficulty you face is that pain has taken control of your steering wheel and is driving you places you don't want to go. The aim of ACT treatment for chronic pain is not to rid yourself of the pain experience, but to get back into the stream of your life. We'll help you learn how to give pain, along with the associated, less-than-pleasant experiences, thoughts, and feelings, space to be with you as you float down that stream.

WHO THIS BOOK IS FOR

This book is for anyone who suffers from chronic pain, anyone with a family member or friend in chronic pain, or professionals who treat people with chronic pain. How you relate to the text will differ depending on which of these groups you fall into.

People with chronic pain: If you suffer from fibromyalgia, general musculoskeletal pain, low back pain, neck and shoulder pain, or any sort of pain that has recurred over a long period of time and has not been remedied by the usual medical treatments, this book is written for you. This workbook will help you to learn about the symptoms of pain, as well as the causes, effects, and standard treatments of pain. Most of all, it will help you learn how to help yourself and reclaim your quality of life. Since the majority of people around the world with chronic pain are women, this book is somewhat oriented toward women, but men are included, too, and will recognize the common aspects and processes of the pain experience.

Family and friends of people in chronic pain: If you're close to someone who suffers from chronic pain, this workbook will help you support your loved one. Understanding the concepts and techniques in this book will give you the opportunity to support your friend or family member on their path to rebuilding a life that is full of value and vitality. Because some of the concepts in ACT may seem a bit strange by traditional Western standards, there are times when people who are being treated with ACT are not fully supported on this path by their loved ones. Reading this book will give you the insight and understanding you need to stand by the person in your life who has chronic pain. And who knows? You may learn something along the way that you can take with you on your own path as well.

Professionals: As a medical professional, whether a psychologist, nurse, physician, occupational therapist, physical therapist, social worker, or alternative therapist, you know it can be difficult to help people with chronic pain. Some of this difficulty is rooted in the type of organization you work for; it may have restrictions in regard to how much time you can allot to patients, as well as what solutions you can offer. In this case, you may want to suggest this workbook to your patients with chronic pain. Additionally, medical professionals working with people with chronic pain run a higher risk of developing chronic stress disorders themselves. When patients are stuck, medical professionals run the risk of getting stuck in a feeling of hopelessness. You're in this profession because you want to help people, and it's frustrating when it seems impossible to do so. Beyond helping your patients with chronic pain, the concepts and processes outlined in this workbook may be of help to you in coping with the demands of your profession.

TAKE A CHANCE

If you've been suffering from chronic pain, what have you got to lose in trying a revolutionary new therapy that has been proven to help people in chronic pain regain their lives? How many therapeutic approaches to pain have you tried at this point? How many of them have worked for you? If you've opened this book, these approaches probably haven't been very effective. But now you have an opportunity to try something new. This way of approaching and understanding your pain may change your perspective, not only on your pain, but on the very way you see yourself as a human being. The ACT approach is revolutionary. It's unlike any other current approaches to dealing with chronic pain. Why not take a chance? After all, if you do what you've always done, you'll get what you've always got. Try something new. Try living beyond your pain.

CHAPTER 1

What Is Pain?
What Is ACT?

If you're reading this book, either you or someone you care about is suffering from chronic pain. Perhaps you have a herniated disc in your back and have had back surgery, but you're still in pain. It may be that you suffer from fibromyalgia and your tender spots never seem to let up. Or perhaps you've experienced an injury of some sort and every few weeks it flares up, causing you intense and excruciating pain.

You've probably been around the block again and again with the medical community. You may have tried painkillers, physical therapy, biofeedback, or any one of a myriad of treatments, all promising to alleviate your symptoms. Nonetheless pain still haunts your life, debilitating you and, worst of all, standing between you and the life you want to live.

How many times have you stayed home from work or other important activities in the last year because the pain was just too much? Did you cancel a vacation you were looking forward to because you were afraid the pain might flare up? Perhaps you're fed up with taking painkillers that make you feel dull and numb. Or maybe you're disgusted with the way that the pain has taken away your vitality and held you back from the life you used to dream of living.

This book offers a way out of the trap your pain has bound you in. The treatment method presented in this book is acceptance and commitment therapy, or ACT (pronounced just like "act"). This new type of psychotherapy has been proven effective for treating a number of psychological disorders (Hayes and Strosahl 2005). It has also been shown to be incredibly effective in helping people who suffer from chronic pain (Dahl, Wilson, and Nilsson 2004).

ACT doesn't promise to keep you from feeling pain. In fact, one of the major tenets of ACT is that it's normal to experience pain and even necessary for survival. It's usually an important message from the body, alerting the brain that something's wrong and needs attention. Suffering, on the other hand, is another matter. ACT draws a distinction between pain and suffering. This book will target the suffering caused by your pain, not the pain itself. Before we tackle that conundrum, let's start with an overview of how pain is typically perceived by the Western medical establishment and how it's most often treated.

AN OVERVIEW OF PAIN

According to the International Association for the Study of Pain, pain is defined as "an unpleasant sensory and emotional experience associated with actual or potential tissue damage, or described in terms of such damage" (Merskey and Bogduk 1994, 210-211). If you look closely at this definition, you'll notice that it includes absolutely nothing that can be measured objectively. Let's deconstruct it in order to develop a better understanding of what's really being said here.

First of all, we're told that "pain is an unpleasant sensory and emotional experience." Anyone who has suffered from any kind of pain can tell you this much. The definition doesn't give us any information about how much unpleasantness constitutes pain. It doesn't even say how much of the sensory information constituting pain is based on physical symptoms versus psychological or emotional issues.

Second, this definition suggests that pain is "associated with actual or potential tissue damage, or described in terms of such damage." This part of the definition tells us that what you're experiencing can be called "pain" even if no real damage has occurred. There can be actual damage, as the definition suggests, or there can be potential damage. But the real kicker is the last phrase, which states that the unpleasant sensory and emotional experience only need be "described in terms of" tissue damage. This means that for the purposes of the International Association for the Study of Pain, there is no definable distinction in the way that pain operates in people who have real injuries and those who don't. This has far-reaching ramifications because most of the pain treatments in Western medicine are based on the association's information.

All this is to say that the totality of Western science's understanding of pain comes down to this simple statement: Pain is an absolutely subjective experience. There are no objective measures by which your pain can be measured. We cannot reliably compare your pain with that of anyone else on the planet. Your pain is yours. And despite any and all efforts to understand it or ameliorate it, it will always remain your subjective experience.

Although your pain is a subjective experience, keep in mind that you're not alone. Pain is one of the most frequent reasons people visit a physician. Next to infectious illness, musculoskeletal pain is the most common symptom seen at primary care centers in the European Union and the United States (Nachemson and Jonsson 2000).

Let's take back pain as an example. This is the most common type of pain complained of in the United States after headaches. At any given time, 15 to 30 percent of the population suffers from back pain, and about 60 to 70 percent of the population will suffer from back pain at some point in their lives (Andersson 1997; Raspe 1993; Skekelle 1997). In a Swedish study, 50 percent of fifteen-year-old children had already experienced back pain (Brattberg 1993, 1994).

None of this is said to give short shrift to the amount of physical pain you may be experiencing right now. Your pain is real. But it may be a comfort to know there are millions of people out there who are also suffering right now. In fact, it could arguably be stated that everyone out there is suffering in one way or another. The concept that everyone is suffering to some degree is the starting point for ACT. However, we need to do a little more investigation into pain before we can go there.

TYPICAL WESTERN TREATMENTS FOR PAIN

Modern Western culture is characterized by a general feel-good orientation that teaches us to avoid pain, suffering, or any other undesirable feeling. You don't have to look far for evidence of this attitude. The airwaves, the print media, and the Internet are littered with the message "Don't put up with pain." Never before in human history have we had so many ways to alleviate, control, or numb pain. What is the result? The number of people who suffer from chronic pain has never been greater. Approximately 50 percent of people on disability in the United States and Europe are unable to work due to chronic musculoskeletal pain (Waddell and Norlund 2000).

Medications

The incredible number of pain medications available to us is a testament to this feel-good attitude. You can walk into your local pharmacy or grocery store and choose any one of hundreds of medications promising to relieve your pain. Of course, prescription medications are more powerful than anything you can get over the counter. And these ultrapowerful pain medications are one of the most common means doctors use to try to help their patients overcome pain. More likely than not, you have been prescribed some type of medicine or multiple medications for your pain.

Several different categories of drugs are prescribed for pain. Although what follows is not a comprehensive overview of these medications, it should give you an idea of what is out there and how effective (or ineffective) these medications are. If you're currently taking pain medications, pay particular attention to the section that discusses the type of medication you're taking.

Analgesic Drugs, or Painkillers

Despite the fact that more people in pain use analgesic drugs than any other treatment method, there are surprisingly very few controlled studies showing their effectiveness. The few studies that have been done only focused on short-term relief of temporary pain. The general recommendation from the review done by the U.S. Agency for Health Care Policy and Research (now the Agency for Healthcare Research and Quality) is that painkillers shouldn't be used in the long run for chronic pain (Bigos et al. 1994). At best, they're ineffective for long-term use, and at worst, they're addictive and have potentially damaging side effects. The review also points out that long-term use of painkillers may, in fact, cause more pain.

Some examples of the most common painkillers that have been evaluated are acetaminophen (brand names include Tylenol and Panadol), codeine, acetylsalicylic acid (more commonly known as aspirin), and dextropropoxyphene (brand names include Darvon and Doloxene).

Nonsteroid Anti-inflammatory Drugs (NSAIDs)

A number of studies have evaluated anti-inflammatory drugs and injections in treatment of chronic pain (for example, Matsumo, Kaneda, and Nohara 1991; Postacchini, Facchini, and Palieri 1988). All have shown that these drugs have little effect on pain in the long run. In fact, some studies indicate that long-term use of NSAIDs can lead to potentially damaging side effects, particularly in the elderly (Van Tulder, Goossens, and Nachemson 2000).

Some of the most common NSAIDs evaluated in the studies above were ibuprofen (brand names include Advil and Midol), piroxicam (brand name Feldene), and diclofenac (brand name Voltaren).

Muscle Relaxants

There is some evidence that muscle relaxants, or benzodiazepines, are effective on pain in the short term (Arbus et al. 1990), but no evidence that long-term use of these drugs is effective for chronic pain. In addition, about 30 percent of patients using muscle relaxants reported side effects (Van Tulder, Goossens, and Nachemson 2000).

The most common muscle relaxants evaluated were orphenadrine (brand names include Norflex), chlormezanone, cyclobenzaprine (brand names include Flexenil), and diazepam (brand names include Valium).

Antidepressants

Antidepressant drugs are prescribed quite frequently for patients with chronic pain. However, none of the studies evaluated by independent government agencies (such as the U.S. Agency for Health Care Policy and Research) showed that antidepressants had any positive effect on either pain or symptoms of depression for patients with chronic pain (Van Tulder, Goossens, and Nachemson 2000).

The most common antidepressant drugs evaluated were trazodone (brand names include Desyrel), imipramine (brand names include Tofranil), and amitriptyline.

Epidural Steroid Injections

There's little evidence that epidural steroid injections, used to reduce inflammation and thus reduce pain, are actually a viable solution for pain problems. While there's some evidence both for and against the effectiveness of these injections for pain in general, most of the studies haven't shown them to reduce pain even in the short term. None of the studies done thus far have shown any positive effects of epidural steroid injections in the long run for people with chronic pain (Kaneda, Matsumo, and Nohara 1991).

The most common epidural steroid injections contained procaine (brand names include Novocain), methylprednisolone (brand names include Medrol), and bupivacaine (brand names include Sensorcaine).

Nondrug Therapies

A number of nondrug therapies are also currently used in the treatment of pain. Most of these are not particularly promising, yielding results similar to those shown above for pain medications. However, there are several nondrug treatments that actually do show positive results. We'll describe a few of these treatments and studies of their effectiveness to give you a better picture of available pain treatments.

Multidisciplinary Pain Treatment

Probably the most common type of treatment for people with chronic pain is a multidisciplinary approach to rehabilitation. Such programs usually consist of a team of specialists focused on different aspects of your pain problem. Included on the team are physicians that specialize in pain, psychologists, physical therapists, occupational therapists. The team often also includes social workers who specialize in helping disabled people get jobs.

A considerable number of studies indicate that this type of multidisciplinary approach does have long-term positive effects for people in chronic pain. Interestingly, most of the success from these treatment programs has been measured in terms of improved quality of life and being able to go back to work (Donaldson et al. 1994; Newton-John, Spence, and Schotte 1995). These studies haven't measured improvement in terms of actual reduction in the patient's physical pain.

These programs are usually five to ten weeks long and require full-time participation by the patient. Components of the program include exercise, physical therapy, ergonomic training, body awareness training, and stress management. No study evaluating these programs has been able to show which of the particular elements included in the programs was effective in helping the patient.

Transcutaneous electric nerve stimulation (TENS)

The TENS treatment method uses electrical stimulation of the nerve endings as a means of reducing pain. This practice is based on a theory that the brain can only process four to five nerve signals through the spinal cord at one time. By sending enough competing information to the brain via the spinal cord, the pain signals are disrupted, diminishing the amount of pain the patient actually feels.

The use of TENS for chronic pain has been evaluated, but the results are contradictory. While some studies showed positive effects on both pain and function, other studies showed no long-term results at all (Hackett, Seddon, and Kaminski 1988; Herman et al. 1994). Consequently, no real conclusions can be drawn as to its effectiveness.

EMG Biofeedback

EMG biofeedback is one treatment for pain you may not have encountered, as it's less common than the others described here. EMG biofeedback aims to tell you how your muscles are working, and specifically whether they're tensed or relaxed at particular times. To achieve this, the patient is hooked up to an electromyogram, an apparatus that provides information (feedback) about how his or her muscles are working. The purpose is usually to give the patient information they can use to learn how to consciously relax at times when their pain flares up. Most of the studies evaluating EMG biofeedback have shown that the technique itself has no positive effects for people with chronic pain (Asfour et al. 1990; Donaldson et al. 1994). However, studies have shown that relaxing can help diminish pain a great deal (Newton-John, Spence, and Schotte 1995).

ANALYZING THE EFFECTIVENESS OF PAIN MANAGEMENT

Before you get started on the book's first exercise, which will help you reflect on your experiences with pain management, we'll take a moment to introduce you to Beth, who also suffers from chronic pain. You'll learn more about her experiences as the book progresses.

■ Beth's Story

Beth, a thirty-three-year-old assistant teacher at an elementary school, loved teaching and helping children grow and learn. It had always been her life's dream to be a schoolteacher, and each day she was in the classroom made her feel she was on a path toward fulfilling that desire. She had planned to go back and finish college many times, both before and after she got married, but her husband was so busy with his career and then the children came. She continued to wait for the right opportunity and never gave up her dream.

Unfortunately, Beth has suffered from chronic pain for the last five years. She had been tense and tired for a number of years previously, trying to be the perfect mom, wife, teacher, daughter, daughter-in-law, sister, and hostess. To keep up with all the demands made on her, she cut corners by not taking care of herself. This came naturally, since her belief was that a good mother, wife, or teacher would put others' needs before her own. One day at school, Beth damaged her rotator cuff while lifting a heavy child from his wheelchair to the toilet. Beth's shoulder became terribly inflamed, and she blamed herself for not using the lift provided.

The pain was excruciating for the first couple of days. After that it turned into a dull roar in the back of her mind, tormenting her every day. Still, she might not have opted to have surgery, but then she started having severe problems with her range of motion. At first she just had a hard time lifting her hand over her head. But as the months passed, eventually she was barely able to lift her arm at all.

Sadly, her real problems started after the surgery. At first it seemed that her shoulder was healed, so she started using it as though nothing had happened. To her surprise and horror, this freedom lasted only a few weeks. Then her pain returned, but now it was worse than before. She couldn't understand what was going on. A number of trips to the doctor resulted only in more confusion and a prescription for Darvon.

When she took the painkillers, her pain was diminished but she had a hard time concentrating. She didn't fully understand that this was happening until parents started complaining to the principal about her and trying to get her fired. At that point, Beth began to see that the painkillers were dulling her mind and making her less effective at the job she loved so much.

EXERCISE: YOUR EXPERIENCE WITH PAIN MANAGEMENT

At this point, take some time to reflect on the pain management strategies discussed above. Which ones have you tried? How effective have they been? Consider their effectiveness in terms of both short-term and long-term pain relief. Also think about what impact these strategies have had on your quality of life. Have they helped you do the things you want to do and live life as you want to? Have they had any negative impacts that have kept you from achieving your goals?

Review all of the types of pain management you've tried. Even if they weren't in the list mentioned above, go ahead and list them so you can get a clear picture of what you've tried so far. Think not only in terms of actual treatment therapies but also about other ways that you've tried to treat yourself. Have you been self-medicating with alcohol or illegal drugs? Have you wasted days watching TV, trying to numb yourself? Think of all the treatments you've received from others, treatments you've tried on yourself, and methods you've used to escape or numb your feelings. List them below, filling in all the columns for each. If you need more space than is provided, feel free to photocopy this worksheet or write your answers in a journal.

Once you've filled in everything you can think of, take a look at the example from Beth, which follows. Reading what she wrote may help you come up with additional items.

Type of pain treatment	Short-term effects on pain	Long-term effects on pain	Long-term effects on quality of life

BETH'S EXPERIENCES WITH PAIN MANAGEMENT

Type of pain treatment	Short-term effects on pain	Long-term effects on pain	Long-term effects on quality of life
Painkillers	Some relief	None	Inhibited my ability to teach.
Surgery	Total relief for a short time	None	Improvement for a while, then the real pain began.
Physical therapy	No real change	None	None. If anything, I was let down because my pain didn't improve.
Watched TV for 3 days once, trying to forget the pain	None	None	None. But in the short term I felt stupid for wasting so much time.
Drinking alcohol to numb myself	Minor improvement for a short time	None	At some point I started waking up every morning feeling sick and having a headache. I knew I was drinking too much.

HOW ACT DIFFERS FROM OTHER TREATMENTS

It may have come as a surprise to you that conventional treatments for chronic pain have yielded such mixed results, especially given all of the glowing advertising, support from the medical industry, media coverage, and popular belief in these treatments. We're not presenting this information to disillusion you about the way the medical establishment works. Nor are we suggesting that you abandon any treatments you're currently pursuing. Decisions of that nature should only be made in conjunction with your doctor. This is especially true of decisions concerning medications, as discontinuing medications without medical supervision can have serious side effects.

That said, it's interesting to note that the research tells a very different story than the one fed to us by the culture at large. The message of every one of the pain therapies mentioned above is simply this: Get rid of the pain. As discussed earlier, in the current feel-good era everything in our culture teaches us that we need to avoid pain at all costs. ACT suggests something radically different. It may be hard for you to accept at first, but stick with it. We think there's a good chance you'll find the payoff to be worth your effort and faith.

Why Avoiding Pain Is the Problem

A great deal of research has proven that avoiding a situation, taking steps to escape from it, or numbing yourself to the feelings brought up by that experience actually makes you more mentally averse to the situation. In ACT, we call this unwillingness to remain in contact with a painful event *experiential avoidance* (Hayes, Strosahl, and Wilson 1999). Perhaps an example will help illustrate this concept.

Let's imagine for a moment that when you were very young you were taught that dogs are dangerous and you were instructed to stay away from them at all costs. Your father was almost killed by a dog when he was young, and both of your parents were terrified that you might be hurt by one as well, so they slapped your hand every time you reached out to pet a dog as you passed it on the street. Now let's imagine that this was taken to an extreme. Your parents got so worried about dogs that they wouldn't even let you have a picture of a dog or a toy dog, and if you but uttered the word "dog" you were slapped—hard. Let's say this went on for years and years. In fact, throughout your entire childhood you were trained to believe that dogs are dangerous and should be avoided at all costs.

Then one day you move out of your parents' house. As an adult, you rationally understand that dogs aren't bad in and of themselves. Do you think you could own one as a pet in this situation? Do you think you could even approach or pet a dog, even a small, friendly one?

The unfortunate answer is that you probably wouldn't be able to do it. You would be so conditioned to fear everything associated with dogs that you wouldn't even be able to think about one without invoking the same psychological response as when you were struck for trying to touch one. You would be afraid, angry, and depressed, thinking that someone was going to strike you even though the possibility of being punished had been removed.

Clearly this is an extreme, possibly even ridiculous example. However, we arbitrarily avoid experiences all the time. Because the example above is a description of some basic premises about the way the mind works, what held true above also applies to virtually any situation where you intentionally or unintentionally avoid experiences of any kind. Over time, you become averse to them, even if they hold no immediate danger for you.

Pain is a perfect example of this. In its basic form, pain is an important set of information. Your body is trying to communicate something to you. When you break your leg, your body generates pain as a signal to let your brain know that something is wrong and that something needs to be done to remedy the situation. Pain in and of itself actually is a good thing.

The problem with chronic pain is that the pain signals never stop. Even if you aren't in immediate danger, the pain signals carry on, and you're conditioned to think you need to do something to stop or change the pain. You're built to think you need to avoid the pain experience, a concept underscored by our culture. And your problem is redoubled by the fact that avoiding your pain causes more pain.

Look at the list of your pain management strategies above. While some of them may have worked in the short term, how many worked in the long term? Probably not many, otherwise you wouldn't be reading this book. But the question is bigger than that. How many of these pain avoidance strategies have forced you to constrain yourself or your life in some way? Do you feel as though your pain has made your life close in around you? Is the act of avoiding pain costing you the life you want to be living?

For Beth this was definitely the case. Taking painkillers inhibited her ability to teach. It also stopped her from going back to college and finishing her degree so that she could pursue the kind of job she really wanted for herself. And not only was her lifelong dream impeded by her attempts to avoid pain, she also felt like a bad mom for not being more available to her children and like a bad wife for not supporting her husband as much as she thought she should. She continuously had a sense of guilt about letting everyone around her down, and she was dangerously close to falling into problems with alcoholism. In her attempts to avoid pain, she simply caused herself additional pain. All the while, the reinforcement she got when her pain avoidance strategies worked in the short term kept her on the path of experiential avoidance.

This pain caused by pain is what we refer to as suffering. As if pain by itself weren't enough . . .

The Difference Between Pain and Suffering

There's an important difference between avoiding dangerous events and avoiding feelings and thoughts about dangerous events. The first is necessary for your survival; the second can seriously handicap your life. It's not always easy to see the difference. When you don't accept your feelings of sadness, uncertainty, or worthlessness elicited by the pain experience, your pain turns into suffering. It's okay to be sad about being sad, be afraid when your body panics, or feel pain when you think about painful experiences. It's when you start doing things to avoid this suffering that you get stuck in chronic pain.

In our experience, most people with chronic pain have altered their life in some way to accommodate their pain. In essence, this is done to avoid the experience of pain. But avoidance of this nature causes suffering, which causes more pain, which causes more suffering (Hayes, Strosahl, and Wilson 1999). This is an endless cycle, drawing people who suffer from chronic pain into a battle they can never win.

This book is designed to help you learn to see the difference between pain and suffering. It will teach you how to break this cycle and keep from getting stuck in chronic pain.

ACCEPT, CHOOSE, AND TAKE ACTION

Is your life in any way inhibited by your pain? We're guessing that your response to this question is yes, otherwise you wouldn't have picked up this book. The difference between ACT and all the other therapies out there comes down to this simple concept: It isn't the pain itself, but your response to the pain that is the problem. We don't believe that getting rid of the pain will change anything. Imagine for a moment that you could get rid of all the pain. What would be different? What would you do? This is possible. There are enough drugs on the market (legal and otherwise) that would numb you from all pain for the rest of your life. But at what cost?

We believe that people in chronic pain are trying to escape the pain so that they can change something in their life and open doors to possibilities their pain has seemed to prevent. You would do something you aren't doing now if you weren't in pain.

What if you were to focus on something other than getting rid of the pain? Why not focus on living your life with the pain? What if that were possible? What would it mean for you? What if you could expand enough to accept your pain and live the life you desire with that pain along for the ride? Indeed, this is precisely what we suggest, and doing so goes to the core of ACT's principles. ACT doesn't just stand for acceptance and commitment therapy. It's an elegant acronym that also serves as a mnemonic for the three simple concepts at the heart of ACT: Accept, Choose, and Take action (Hayes, Strosahl, and Wilson 1999).

Accept

If experiential avoidance is the root of your suffering, its counterpart is acceptance. Acceptance is the act by which you allow yourself to willingly engage your pain. It is indeed possible to learn to accept your pain and abandon the fight against it. Thousands of people treated for chronic pain using ACT have been successful in doing this. So although it isn't an easy thing to do and in fact is fairly tricky, it is doable. The portions of this book on mindfulness, letting go of control, and learning to hear your thoughts for what they are instead of what they say they are will help you learn how to accept your pain instead of fighting against it.

Choose

Once you learn to accept your pain and live with it, rather than in opposition to it, you are free to choose how you want to live. Imagine this is possible for you. What would you do? Be assured, this is possible for you and you can live the life you want to live; you simply need to learn how. Though it isn't quite as straightforward to do as it may sound, with a little work you can learn to choose the life you want to live, rather than allowing the pain to choose for you. This book will help you develop a life compass, a way of discovering your values and determining your direction. The life compass will be your guidepost to the life you choose to lead.

Take Action

What's holding you back from embarking down the road you want to follow? Once you've made a choice about how you want to live, the only thing left to do is to figure out what steps are necessary to get where you want to go. The portion of this book on setting goals will help you develop a structured, step-by-step plan for moving in that direction and achieving a life rich with meaning.

WHERE DO YOU GO FROM HERE?

We believe the tools in this book can help you establish a different kind of life for yourself—one that's based on the way you want to live rather than the way your pain tells you to live. But like all changes, this will take time and effort on your part. The rest of this book is organized to help you start on a path toward accepting your pain and living a life you value. It will give you a step-by-step model you can follow to start unraveling the riddles of your suffering.

Think of it as a journey. Sometimes the road will seem straightforward; other times you'll be confused at the twists and turns it takes. The road has many bumps and potholes. You may climb steep hills or descend into deep valleys. Stick with it. We believe you'll find fresh air and a beautiful sunrise at the end of it.

In the next chapter we'll help you begin to distinguish more clearly between pain and suffering (Hayes, Strosahl, and Wilson 1999), or what we will call "clean pain" versus "dirty pain." You'll also start to learn about the paradoxical nature of control.

CHAPTER 2

Controlling Your Pain
Is Not the Answer

As mentioned in chapter 1, ACT draws a distinction between pain and suffering. The ACT argument is that it's not your pain that causes your problems, but the way you suffer as a result of your pain. Therefore, the goal of the treatment is not the reduction of pain, but the elimination of suffering. Let us be clear that we are not promising to eliminate your pain. That may be impossible. But we can offer to help you change your perspective on pain to such a degree that the effects of pain on your life will change substantially, and for the better.

The key to this whole suffering business comes down to one word: control. Everything in our culture teaches us that our happiness relies on our ability to control our experiences and extinguish pain from our existence. This undoubtedly sounds like an attractive option if you've been suffering from physical pain for years on end. And it's not just our feel-good culture that teaches us we need to get rid of pain, it's the entire Western medical establishment. All of the common treatments for pain discussed in chapter 1 have a single purpose: to control pain. The message all around us seems to be "If you aren't controlling the pain, the pain is controlling you." So you've worked diligently to control the pain. You've made choices you wouldn't otherwise make in order to keep the pain at bay. You take medications that may or may not keep that pain monster away, even though those medications may create other problems. You control, control, control until you've controlled yourself into a corner. At that point, who is really in control? At what point do your attempts to control the pain actually give the pain control over you?

It may even be that your attempts to control your pain are exacerbating your frustration with your life. How much time have you spent trying to ameliorate your pain that you would have liked to spend other ways? How much effort have you put into your less-than-successful attempts to control pain? Wouldn't you rather have dedicated that effort to other pursuits? How do the medications make you feel? How well is this control business really working?

What if there's another approach that you haven't conceived of up to this point? What if letting go of control were an option? What if you could just let go of your end of the rope in this tug-of-war with pain?

THE SERENITY CREED

We want to be clear that ACT is not a nihilistic philosophy. We're not telling you to simply give up and accept a life of misery. What we're suggesting is subtler than that. The ACT approach is encapsulated nicely in the well-known serenity creed: Grant me the courage to change the things I can, the serenity to accept the things I cannot change, and the wisdom to know the difference.

Many of you are undoubtedly already familiar with the serenity creed. It's found everywhere these days, from offices to church meeting rooms; on plaques, jewelry, candles, and wind chimes; and marketed to specific groups ranging from nurses to golfers. Though it's so ubiquitous in our culture that we may tend not to read or think about what it's saying anymore, its widespread popularity indicates that it speaks to people at a very deep level.

Looking more closely at this popular prayer is illuminating. One of the things it tells us is that there are things we cannot change. Indeed, we know this to be true in the outer world, but what if it also holds true for our inner experience, including pain? There is little doubt you have tried hard to change your experience with pain. You've probably engaged in many different pain management strategies. Perhaps there are simply some aspects of your pain that you can't change. If that turns out to be true, what can you do with the part of your pain that isn't reparable?

Of course, there are aspects of your pain that can be changed or managed. You've already been working on these. It's worthwhile to continue doing so as long as it's not at the expense of living your life. For the most part, human beings are good at solving problems. When there's work to be done, we know what to do. And pain is a good motivator, so you probably already know how to fix the parts of your pain that are fixable. But when your quest for a pain-free existence takes over your life, there's a problem. When your battle with pain keeps you home from work, or school, or whatever else you want to be doing, hasn't the pain won? What then? When you run up against the part of your pain that you haven't been able to repair, what's to be done? This is the part of our experience where human beings tend to have more problems. We hope to help you answer some of these questions for yourself as you proceed through the book. We believe the answers are wrapped up in the words that describe ACT: acceptance and commitment.

One thing is certain: The more you struggle to fix what cannot be fixed, the more you suffer. If you are suffering with chronic pain, we posit that the portion of your suffering driven by the pain itself is actually quite small. Your efforts to control your experience of pain are what drives the majority of your suffering. This is because most efforts at control are based on restricting your life or yourself in some way. For example, imagine a friend stops by and asks you if you want to go out for a walk. It's a lovely day, the sun is out but it's not too hot, the birds are singing, and you can smell spring in the air. Unfortunately you can also feel that aching pain in your lower back that never seems to go away. Today the pain is actually fairly bad. It's been aching since you woke up and you feel tormented by it. You want to go for the walk, but you're worried that doing so might exacerbate the problem and make your pain unbearable. So you tell your friend that you're going to pass on the walk because your back is bothering you. Your friend understands, wishes you well, and leaves. What has changed in regard to your pain? Nothing. But your life has been diminished in some small way by losing that opportunity. This may not seem like such a problem if you make such choices only occasionally. But what happens if you build your life on these choices?

What this comes down to is a problem with the control paradigm. You think you can control your pain by not going on the walk. But after choosing not to walk, you're still left with the pain. So you make more and more choices of this nature, hoping that diminishing the possibilities for creating more pain will make you feel less pain. As the battle to control your pain continues, your life becomes progressively smaller and smaller—closing in around you. Because you're sold on your control strategies, you fight harder and harder, but all the while you feel less and less alive. Days, weeks, months, or years later you still have the pain, with the added burden of a life that's no longer fulfilling for you. Does this sound like a familiar pattern?

This type of suffering basically stems from an inability to accept the things you cannot change. Later in the book we'll devote a lot of attention to helping you learn how to accept. For now, let's look more closely at the last line of the serenity creed and explore the wisdom to know the difference between that which you can change and that which you cannot change. Learning to make this distinction will allow you to decide when to apply the acceptance skills we'll teach you and when you have the choice to act to change your experience.

Learning to Know the Difference

There's a kind of dividing line between where pain ends and the suffering your pain causes you begins. This same line marks the difference between the aspects of your pain experience that you have control over and the ones you don't. ACT draws this line between the physical pain you feel and the way pain is interrupting or inhibiting your life, understanding them as two different kinds of pain. We call the first one "clean pain." It's a simple, immediate, physical sensation that tells us something's wrong. An aching back, the sore wrists of carpal tunnel syndrome, tender spots, an old ankle injury that flares up regularly—these things are all clean pain.

What we call "dirty pain" is something quite different. Dirty pain is all the reactions you have to your physical pain (Hayes, Strosahl, and Wilson 1999). Dirty pain is the things your mind tells you about your physical pain. It's the epithets that run through your head when you do something that puts you in pain. It's the avoidance behaviors you engage to keep yourself from feeling pain. Dirty pain is your attempts to relieve yourself of pain where relief may not be possible.

Clean pain is just pain. Dirty pain is all the stuff that goes along with your pain. Dirty pain is where pain itself ends and suffering begins. Dirty pain is your attempts to control that which cannot be controlled, your attempts to fix that which cannot be repaired. Clean pain is a vital hum and a valuable messenger that comes along with existing in this world. Dirty pain is the muck you get mired in trying to silence that hum. Clean pain is rooted in the part of your pain you have little control over. Working on your dirty pain, however, will prove to be very fruitful. It's ironic that people who suffer from chronic pain are usually trying to do the opposite. They attempt to control their clean pain while letting their dirty pain run rampant. This is a mistake. It's a mistake that's reinforced by nearly everything we know, but it's a mistake nonetheless.

By this point, we've established that you can't eliminate pain. But don't just believe what you read here (never a good idea), look at your own experience. We think you'll come to the same conclusion if you're honest about your situation.

But you can substantially reduce your suffering. To do so, you need to look at the way your dirty pain operates and unravel yourself from its tentacles. Dirty pain usually comes in three different forms: mental scripts, avoidance behaviors, and what we call "values illness."

Mental Scripts

Mental scripts are the thought processes that play out when you have a reaction to your pain experience. When you learn to watch for them (which you will in the mindfulness component of this book), you'll notice there are quite a lot of them. Here are some examples:

- Searching for reasons you're in pain. (You might say something to yourself like "I told you not to lift that by yourself; you know what happens when you aren't careful" or "You're a bad person and deserve to be in pain.")

- Yelling epithets at yourself in your head. ("You hopeless idiot! Why can't you just do what I tell you!")

- Reciting rules you've established for yourself around your pain. (For example, you might think "When I get too tired, I end up in pain.")

These are only a few of the ways mental scripts might present themselves. Essentially, mental scripts are all the things you tell yourself about your pain experience. If you climb a ladder, fall, and hurt yourself, you might say, "If only I hadn't done that, I wouldn't be in pain." True or not (and there is much debate about that), this is a mental script.

Avoidance Behaviors

Avoidance behaviors, which encompass anything you do, avoid, or avoid doing so as not to feel pain, are particularly dangerous. Extensive research has shown that experiential avoidance (the act of avoiding a particular experience due to some feared outcome) doesn't reduce pain; it actually *increases* pain (Gutiérrez et al. 2004).

Perhaps you have some experience of what avoidance does in other areas of your life. You may have been in a car accident that gave you a real scare, and afterward everything in your body and mind told you that driving a car is dangerous. You probably felt hesitant to get into your car and start driving again. You may have only had minor tissue damage from the accident itself, but the whole incident made you scared and stiff. Since you need to drive your car, you probably went ahead and started driving again even though your mind was yelling at you not to do it. It may be that your driving has changed, and you're much more cautious now. You may see and feel danger all around you that you didn't see or feel before the accident. You might override these scary thoughts and feelings and continue driving, or you might yield to what these thoughts and feelings are telling you and start to avoid certain activities that involve driving.

In essence, experiential avoidance is an inability to accept some thought or feeling that consequently causes you to avoid a particular circumstance or event (Hayes, Strosahl, and Wilson 1999). The funny thing about experiential avoidance is that it often becomes automatic and we end up forgetting why we started avoiding the experience in the first place. We even create logical reasons for our avoidance behavior. For example, someone who's afraid of elevators may tell you that she prefers the stairs for exercise. Someone who's afraid of going to work and ending up in more pain might say he doesn't like his job, even though that isn't an accurate assessment of the situation. To be able to get to where you want to go, you'll need to look more carefully at what you're avoiding that's associated with your pain. We'll explore this topic throughout the book, but you can get started a little later in this chapter with the worksheet on clean pain versus dirty pain.

Avoidance behaviors specific to chronic pain take on many forms. Here are just a few examples of avoidance behaviors you may engage in:

- Using medications to avoid pain entirely rather than just dampen it enough to live your life

- Refusing to engage in certain activities because they will or may cause you pain

- Settling for less than what you really want because you believe your pain rules out those possibilities

- Dissociating from yourself so as not to feel the pain

Avoidance behaviors are incredibly seductive. They look like the answer. They look like a means to control your experience. Our whole Western culture and the health care system proffer a wide variety of avoidance strategies as the answers to your pain problems and suggest these can ultimately lead to your happiness. There is very little said about the opposite. In reality, pain is a natural part of living, and we grow and develop by practicing tolerance and acceptance of negative feelings in order to go forward in life.

Most of us admire people like Nelson Mandela, Christopher Reeve, or Rosa Parks—people who have shown incredible endurance of pain and suffering in order to pursue their vision of making a meaningful contribution to the world. That is the choice all of us make every minute of every day. You can take steps down a path that's vital and meaningful to you if you wish to. This may mean bringing pain with you, but it may just be worth it if the alternative is a more confined life. Choosing the path of experiential avoidance may be less painful for you in the short term, but it will ultimately shut you into a life that's increasingly constricted.

˙Values Illness

In this book, we use "values illness" to describe opting for experiential avoidance and moving away from the life you want to live. It's a little hard to explain, since we've not yet fully outlined what we mean by values (we'll do that in chapter 3), but it's important for you to have a basic grasp of this concept early on.

Everyone has dreams for their life and certain goals. There are particular things or people or ways of being that you value. In this context, "value" doesn't imply a religious ethic; rather, we mean value in the sense of deeming something to be of relative worth or importance. There are many things you might value, and to live a valued life is to live in a way that's meaningful for you, to move in the direction you most deeply want to move in, and to not be stopped by perceived hindrances. Values illness is the antithesis of a valued life. If you're suffering from values illness, you may have noticed some of these symptoms:

- Giving up on a higher education because you're afraid the pain will keep you from being able to concentrate

- Quitting a job you'd always dreamed of due to the pain it caused you

- Deciding against having a family because parenting could be difficult if you're in pain

- Giving up on the idea of a holistic lifestyle because you need pain medications just to get by

These are only a few symptoms of values illness. If your pain has caused you to make substantial concessions in regard to the way you want to live, then you are suffering from values illness.

We'll look at values illness and what you can do about it throughout the rest of this book. In fact, a primary goal of ACT in all contexts is to help people heal from values illness. For now, just think about how values illness may be contributing to your dirty pain. Doing this will take you one step toward healing from it. To help you understand values illness, let's take a look at Eric's situation.

■ Eric's Story

Eric is a carpenter. He's always loved working with tools and building things. It started as a hobby, but when his friends and his wife commented on what beautiful cabinets he made for their living room, he decided to try to turn it into a business. He did and the results were spectacular. In no time at all he became a successful cabinetmaker. He had clients in different parts of the state and even flew across the country from time to time to build things for people who had heard about his beautiful work.

Soon he decided to expand his business beyond cabinetmaking, and eventually he made furniture, beautiful Japanese-style shoji screens, and more. In fact, Eric was considered something of a genius in the world of finish carpentry.

The problems started when he bent over to lift a heavy piece of oak for a project he was working on. He lifted with his back, not his legs. He knew better, but he was in a hurry and didn't care at the time. He's been sorry for that mistake ever since. As he lifted the piece of oak, he heard a small pop in his lower back. At the time he had no idea what had happened. He just felt a sharp, excruciating pain shoot up his spine. He dropped the beautiful oak, which cracked as it hit the floor, and he wasn't able to straighten his back.

A week in bed, a chiropractic appointment, and a prescription for painkillers made some difference . . . for a while. He got back to work, but found himself afraid because of the injury in his back. He watched himself ceaselessly and wondered what good he was as a carpenter without a strong back to support the weight of his work.

After two months he injured his back again and repeated the cycle of a week in bed, chiropractic, and painkillers. But this time he threw out his back again just three days later. This happened several times over the course of two years until he finally decided to give up his carpentry business. The impacts didn't stop there. Many aspects of his life were affected. Not only did he give up a career he really loved, he also started fighting with his wife because he was unhappy and even started drinking pretty heavily.

He went to back specialists, who recommended surgery. He went to physical therapists; they said stretching would be the answer. He tried biofeedback. He had tried just about everything when he decided to see a therapist. By chance, he chose someone who was an ACT practitioner. Although Eric's story up to this point revolves around a life of disappointments due to his struggle with pain, take heart; both Eric and Beth experienced substantially improved quality of life through ACT. Eric's therapist helped him with a program very much like the one in this book. One of the first things the therapist asked him to do was fill out a clean and dirty pain diary, just like the one you'll fill out in the next exercise.

EXERCISE: CLEAN AND DIRTY PAIN DIARY

To help you understand the differences between clean and dirty pain more directly, we ask that you keep a diary of your pain experiences. Use this diary to track how the clean, purely physical pain functions and how the dirty pain functions.

Photocopy the form below and fill it out for at least the next week. (After the week is up, you may find it helpful to continue keeping this diary.) Throughout the coming week, make an entry on the form any time you experience pain. Record all five elements the form covers: note the situation or activity you were engaged in when the pain occurred; describe the physical pain sensation (the kind of clean pain you felt); rate that pain on a scale of 0 to 10; describe your reactions to the pain experience (your dirty pain); and rate your level of suffering because of the dirty pain on a scale of 0 to 10.

	Clean Pain		Dirty Pain	
Situation	Pain description	Level	Pain description	Level

ERIC'S CLEAN AND DIRTY PAIN DIARY

Situation	Clean Pain Pain description	Level	Dirty Pain Pain description	Level
Tried to lift a fairly light hollow door to hang in the kitchen	*Sharp pain in my back*	*7*	*Start thinking about how I gave up my carpentry practice.*	*10*
Tripped on a sweater my wife threw on the bedroom floor	*Light twinge in my back*	*4*	*Start cursing aloud about what a lazy bitch my wife is, even though I don't mean it. She hears me and leaves the room crying.*	*9*
Went for a long ride in the car	*Stiff back when I get out*	*2*	*Start thinking, "Man, I can't even take a damned ride in the car. Well, there's another thing I'll have to watch out for."*	*6*
Bent over to pick up the remote control	*Same old ache*	*5*	*Pop a pill and have a drink so I can watch some TV. I hate it cause I never used to take pills before.*	*8*

THE PAIN CHAIN

Hopefully the exercise above helped you begin to see the difference between your clean pain and your dirty pain. The rest of this book will explore how you can make use of that distinction and how you can ameliorate your suffering (not your pain) by undermining your dirty pain.

One of the worst aspects of dirty pain is that it starts to develop into what we call "the pain chain." In the description of dirty pain above, we suggested that dirty pain manifests itself in three different ways: mental scripts, avoidance behaviors, and values illness. Perhaps it wouldn't be too harmful if your suffering only manifested itself in one of these ways at a time. If you say to yourself, "Damn! I should have been more careful," and that's the end of the story, there would be some harm, but not that much. Unfortunately, when pain's involved, a simple mental script is seldom the end of the story. The real problems occur because the different types of dirty pain lead from one to another, creating a chain of pain that wraps itself around you, binding you and restricting your life.

For those with chronic pain, the complete manifestation of suffering usually happens in about four steps:

1.   Your actual physical pain sensation

2.   The way your mind reacts to this pain

3.   Avoidance or escape behaviors based on what your mind says

4.   Long-term choices based on avoidance and escape behaviors

The first step is clean pain, a simple physical sensation that, if left to its own devices, would cause you some difficulty but wouldn't destroy your life. You'll notice that the remaining steps correspond exactly with the three manifestations of dirty pain—mental scripts, avoidance behaviors, and values illness—each leading to the next until your long-term, life-determining choices are based on pain rather than on what you want out of life. Let's reconsider Eric's story and his pain diary to get a clearer idea of how the pain chain works.

Eric had a career that he really loved—carpentry. After his first experience with back pain, he started having some doubts about himself in the workshop, and we mentioned that Eric watched his back ceaselessly. It's not hard to imagine what this might entail. It's likely he was always telling himself to be careful. Perhaps he was thinking, "I better not lift this too quickly, otherwise I'll end up in pain" or "Maybe I should hold off on finishing that table until tomorrow. I'd like to get it done, but I don't want to injure myself again."

It would be one thing if he thought this and decided to finish the table anyway. But as you know, it doesn't end there. When Eric started avoiding certain tasks to keep himself out of pain, that's when the real suffering began. The point at which Eric decided to restrict his activities based on his back was a fairly slippery slope. Soon enough he was conditioning himself to avoid activities as a means of avoiding pain. In the end he decided to give up his career because the pain was "just too much." Losing his career was such a blow that it led to fighting with his wife, drinking heavily, and taking pills he didn't believe in. One step in the pain chain led to the next, until Eric felt as though his life had been destroyed. Initial thoughts about difficulties with pain led to small avoidance behaviors. Unchecked, these ballooned into a pattern of avoidance in attempts to prevent pain, until finally the pain chain completed itself and he was restricted to a life he no longer enjoyed.

Perhaps this example seems a little extreme to you, but haven't you made similar decisions based on your pain? How much have you lost because pain got in your way? It may be that you've sacrificed more to your pain than you're even aware of right now. Dirty pain is an insidious little monster that creeps up stealthily and can take you by surprise. You don't think you're making decisions on behalf of the pain, but when you start to analyze it you may find that it has taken up more of your life than you had realized.

It's a little like finding a tiger cub in your kitchen. This cute, furry little guy nips at you from time to time when he's hungry. To keep him from nipping at you (after all, the nips *do* hurt), you feed him a nice steak. But every time you feed the little bugger, he grows a little bit. And every time he grows, he demands a little more steak. After feeding him long enough, you have a full-grown tiger on your hands, and he's liable to eat you for dinner instead of the tender steaks you've been feeding him. In the end you can hardly move through your kitchen without getting a leg or arm bit off by this hungry beast.

Does your life feel a little like this? If so, it's because you've been feeding the tiger; you've been encouraging the pain chain to grow. If you want to stop feeding that ravenous creature, you first need to understand how you're feeding it in the first place. The following exercise should shed some light on this.

EXERCISE: THE PAIN CHAIN

After completing your clean and dirty pain diary for a week, take another week and follow the decisions you make based on your pain. When you find yourself making even the smallest concession for your pain (like waiting until your pain subsides to go to the store), note it on the worksheet in the appropriate space. Since you'll probably need to fill out a few of these, make several photocopies of the worksheet rather than filling in the one in the book.

Once you note a decision based on pain avoidance, analyze it and see if you can find the different manifestations of dirty pain that are wrapped up in this decision. If you jotted down "I chose not to go to the store until the pain subsided," you would follow this by trying to remember any mental scripts that led you to this decision (for example, "I can't handle going out today"). Then note the specific avoidance behavior you're engaging in (in this case "not going to the store"). Finally, check in with yourself about any values illness this might reveal. (If this component seems difficult, it can wait until you've read chapter 3, on values.) If you have trouble with this exercise, take a look at the example from Eric, which follows.

Keep in mind that the exercise is not a yardstick for failure; it doesn't record how you're lacking. Its goal is simply to help you unveil what is going on for you. Also note that you need not come to any conclusions about what the exercise tells you at this point. There's plenty of time for that later on.

Decision made based on pain: _____

_____

_____

Mental scripts on which this decision was based: _____

_____

_____

Specific avoidance behavior: _____

_____

_____

Values illness: _____

_____

_____

ERIC'S PAIN CHAIN

Decision made based on pain:

I decided not to purchase the hinges for the kitchen door my wife asked me to hang.

Mental scripts on which this decision was based:

I can't lift the damned door anyway, so why the hell bother with the hinges. I'm such a failure as a husband.

Specific avoidance behavior:

Not going to the store because of pain.

Values illness:

The whole event just reminds me of my old career. I enjoyed building and fixing things so much and I was so good at it. Now I can't even hang a door. Pain has wrecked me.

CREATIVE HOPELESSNESS: A POSITIVE SURRENDER

What we're suggesting in this chapter is actually fairly simple: Control is not the answer. We haven't offered you anything to replace control yet, but we will. In the meanwhile, surrendering to this idea that control may not be possible is a powerful place to be. Have you ever come to a point in your struggle with pain where you simply said, "I can't fix this"? What did that feel like? You may have experienced some grief, but wasn't there also a certain freedom?

You've probably had many experiences of being let down by new "cures" that never pan out. You may even feel that you've been taken for a fool. Perhaps you feel that this is your own fault. At this point you probably have mixed feelings about even trying to regain a life that you value. You've had a lot of experience feeling hopeless and worrying that all of the failed strategies and broken promises about getting rid of your pain are just more evidence that it isn't possible. But some part of you probably feels hopeful about finding solutions so that you can get on with your life. You want to believe there's a way out of your suffering, but you've yet to find any proof of this.

This sense of hopelessness isn't a pleasant feeling, but what if there's actually hope to be found in your feelings and thoughts of hopelessness? You may even feel a little empty, but isn't that emptiness pregnant with possibility? In ACT we call this "creative hopelessness" (Hayes, Strosahl, and Wilson 1999). People are often turned off by the word "hopelessness." It sounds like giving up. So let's look at what we mean by creative hopelessness.

We define creative hopelessness as a place where new possibilities for changing your life arise. You may feel hopeless in the face of this fight with your pain, a fight you haven't been able to win. Since you can't "beat" your pain, what is left for you to do? Giving up is not the answer to this question. Exploring new, uncharted possibilities is what's called for. We encourage people to creatively engage with their lives to find solutions to seemingly hopeless situations.

You may wonder if you'll be overwhelmed by your pain if you relax your control. Since you've explored other solutions and still find yourself in pain, why not try it and find out? Let go a little and follow this path a little further with us. We've helped many others with chronic pain, and we'd like to help you, too.

At this point, you probably have a lot of questions. You may not fully accept the material we've presented in this chapter: that controlling pain isn't the answer; that your suffering is distinct from your pain; and that mental scripts, avoidance behaviors, and values illness, all of which fuel your suffering, compound one another and are what's really restricting your life. If you're having trouble believing in this approach, we encourage you to test it for yourself. The only marker by which any of this work makes sense is your own experience. If it doesn't resonate with you, perhaps it isn't for you. But don't come to that conclusion before you give the ACT approach a try. Stick with it. As you work forward, we'll answer many of the questions you may have. Perhaps what you find will be valuable for you. What have you got to lose?

CHAPTER 3

What Do You Value?

If managing or controlling your pain isn't the answer, then what is? This is the most pressing question for most of our clients when introduced to the idea that pain management may not be the answer they need. Ultimately, the answer is up to you. Though we can't answer this question for you, what we can do is provide you with a model you can use to figure out that answer for yourself. In this chapter, we'll help you explore your values, because that's where the answer lies. If you give it a chance, this just may be the alternative you've been looking for.

You've been fighting a battle with your pain. Over time this battle has started to consume your life. The time you've spent searching for solutions to your pain has likely left you exhausted, stressed-out, and, worst of all, still in pain. You are probably so tired of the pain and so wrapped up in getting rid of it that you've forgotten why you wanted to get rid of it in the first place. So many battles end up this way. The participants are so involved with the fight, they forget why they started fighting to begin with. At first glance, asking you why you want to get rid of your pain may seem like a ridiculous question. Isn't it self-evident? We're suggesting you look at it from a different perspective. Take a moment to stop and ask yourself this question: If I had no pain, what would I do with my life?

What you would do with your life may be the very thing that's been overlooked in your long battle with pain. What if you could learn to do those things *with* your pain? This may sound a bit radical, but what if you could carry your pain with you while you live the life you want to live?

That's what this book is all about: learning to carry your pain with you while pursuing the things that matter to you. Later we'll offer you some concrete strategies for learning how to carry your pain. But right now, let's find out what it is you've been wanting to do all this time.

VALUING: A MEANINGFUL WAY OF LIFE

Values are what bring meaning to your life. Anything you care about deeply is a reflection of your values. They are the basis of how you choose to live your life, and they define the direction you want to go (Hayes, Strosahl, and Wilson 1999). In order to understand this clearly, there are a number of distinctions that need to be made.

The Difference Between Reasons and Choices

ACT is founded on *relational frame theory*, a scientifically based theory about the way human language and cognition work (Hayes 2004). The basic premise of relational frame theory is that human behavior is governed largely through networks of verbally constructed rules, or *relational frames*. While there's no need for a full exploration of relational frames here, it is necessary that you understand certain principles of this theory so that you can completely understand what values are.

Human beings are great rule makers. It's one of the things that's made us the dominant species on the planet. We have the ability, through language, to learn without direct experience. Take, for example, a mother telling her child not touch the hot stove or else the child will be burned. This is a basic "if-then" statement. If you touch the stove, then you'll be burned. Although this may seem pretty basic, it's actually incredibly sophisticated. We are the only species on the planet we know of that has such complex language capabilities. Other animals understand these kinds of causal relationships only through direct experience. A cat won't touch something that's hot twice, but it needs to do it once before it gets the hint. A child need never touch a hot stove to learn it can burn him or her.

In the outside world this is a tool beyond compare (as evidenced by the aforementioned dominance of the human species). However, in our internal world it has some downsides. The problem with this type of rule making, particularly when it comes to something like living with chronic pain, is that it can restrict your life in some very fundamental ways. For example, Eric, whom you met in the previous chapter, developed a rule that when he lifted heavy things, he threw his back out. If he believes this rule and follows it invariably, it means he'll never lift anything heavy again. Though this is a restriction, it may not seem so bad if it keeps him out of pain.

The real problems lie in the ramifications the rule has on the rest of his life. Remember, Eric was a carpenter and loved his work. Carpenters often have to lift heavy things. If he can't do that, how much of a carpenter can he be? Thus, the consequences of applying this rule inflexibly are quite severe. Being a carpenter was one of the most meaningful aspects of his life. And in fact, his life kind of fell apart when he decided he couldn't keep working as a carpenter because of his pain. It would be an exaggeration to say the single rule about lifting heavy things ruined his life, but it certainly contributed to his problems.

It's likely you've experienced something similar. You've probably developed rules for yourself that restrict your life, diminish your vitality, and bar you from doing things that are meaningful to you. Perhaps you've decided that you can't go to the store without taking a painkiller just in case. Or worse, maybe you, like Eric, have abandoned something you cherished because it "caused" the pain. These rules your mind makes can be quite treacherous. Rules limit your flexibility. If, based on your pain, you develop rules that limit your choices, you're left with very little room to live the kind of life you want to live. You may think you're doing this to keep yourself out of pain, but as we explored in chapter 2, this attempt is futile. Avoiding important life experiences in the hope of avoiding pain quickly leads to suffering, redoubling the pain you started with. This is one of the reasons control doesn't work.

Reasons are another kind of rule. Reasons tell us why we do something. Let's look at Sara's situation. She's the mother of three children. She loves them very much and wants to be the best mother she can be to them. The problem is that she has chronic neck pain, and when it acts up she doesn't feel as engaged with them as she'd like to be. When asked why she wants her pain to go away, she answers, "Because I want to be an engaged mother and spend quality time with my children. I don't feel I can do that when I'm in pain." This reason is a judgment Sara has made based on something she desires. She thinks that being pain free will allow her to spend more quality time with her children. But this reasoning implicitly establishes another rule: that the way to be able to spend quality time with her kids is to get rid of her pain. According to that rule, if she doesn't get rid of her pain, she can't spend time with her kids. As you can see, reasons themselves can be a dangerous trap.

But what of the desire behind the reason, where does that come from? If you could get past the reason to the fundamental place that leads you to that reason in the first place, where would you be? This may sound like psychobabble or some bizarre philosophical line of questioning, but bear with it for a moment and see where it takes you.

Most people know or have seen children who ask questions incessantly. There are kids out there who ask why about everything. Often these children follow this course of questioning to a point where there is no longer a way to answer the question. Why does a zebra have stripes? Why is the sky blue? Why is the earth round? Think about a child like that for a moment. If you were once that child yourself, get in contact with that part of yourself once again.

Now think about something that's meaningful to you. Anything at all will do. Then, from the mind frame of that inquisitive child, ask yourself why that thing is meaningful to you. If you come up with an answer, ask the question again. Then do it again. Keep asking the question until you a find a place where you have no answer. If you apply yourself, you will eventually come to the place where there is no longer an answer to your question. Your mind can no longer produce adequate reasons and you are left with some "isness." You appreciate something because you appreciate it. Ultimately, that's what it comes down to. There is a place beyond which reasons cannot be generated.

In considering what you value, eventually you simply make a choice. You can't reason values out. It doesn't work that way. Let's look back at Sara's example for further clarification.

In Sara's case, the choice is to be an engaged mother. This may not sound at all like a choice to you, but in fact it is. Why would she want to be an engaged mother? If you can come up with an answer for this question, that's still just a reason; there's still a deeper level at which you can no longer answer the question.

This place is where your values lie. Values are not based on reasons, they're based on choices. In ACT, we define values as chosen life directions. There are many reasons to be an engaged parent. And if you try, you can probably also find some reasons *not* to be an engaged parent. Either way, if you choose that as a value, the reasons themselves are irrelevant. So here's our first clue as to what values are: They are choices we make about what we want our lives to be about.

Values Are Not Goals

Values and goals are two very different things (Hayes, Strosahl, and Wilson 1999). Both are important, and both will be essential to the work you're doing in this book. Let's look at how they differ.

Goals are practical, obtainable outcomes that you plan for and that you believe move you in valued directions. Goals are stepping-stones that lead you down the path of a valued life. They're distinct from values in that they are the objectives of a valued life. If your values are a compass that points you in the direction you want to go in life, then goals are the waypoints on the map, places you plan to visit as you move in the direction of your values.

Let's explore this using Sara's situation. Sara values being an engaged mother. The means by which she chooses to do this are her goals. Spending more quality time with her children may be a goal Sara has in order to move down the path of being an engaged mother. She may also set many other goals in order to be an engaged mother. Going to soccer games and school plays, checking on her kids' homework after school, taking them to the zoo on the weekends—these are all ways she might express her value of being an engaged mother in a practical way. These types of planned practical manifestations of a person's values are goals.

Your goals should always be judged against your own values, not against what the culture you live in does, what the people around you think, or even what some programmed sense of right and wrong tells you to do. If you set a goal and take a step in a particular direction, you need to check in and see if that step makes you feel vital and alive. If it does, great. If it doesn't, then you should reexamine the goal and see whether or not it's really taking you in the direction you want to go.

In this light, it is often not the activities themselves that are the goals, but the quality of those activities. If Sara wants to be an engaged mother, she might physically sit at her child's soccer match, while her mind is in a totally different place, like planning what to do the next day. She may even end up resenting attending the game because she feels like there are other things she could and should be doing instead.

Sara probably believes that engaged moms go to soccer games because that's what society tells her to believe. She feels she should be at the soccer game even if she doesn't want to be there. But maybe there are ways she can be an engaged mother without going to the soccer game if that doesn't feel like the right thing to do. In fact, planning the next day may be her way of being an engaged mom. It all comes down to personal perspective guided by values.

Goals can help you physically move in your valued direction, but in order to get back your quality of life, you need to judge the quality, the vitality, of each activity against your values. In some cases you may find that what seemed like a worthy goal doesn't advance your sense of vitality. In that case, you may need to adjust your course. Keep in mind that these adjustments are also steps on your valued path as long as you keep your values in your sights.

Without a plan on how to move in a particular direction, you're unlikely to go anywhere at all. This is why goals are so important. Setting goals allows you to establish a game plan for the way you want your values to be expressed in your life. That doesn't necessarily mean the plan will always pan out as you dream it will. Goals can shift and change over time, and they often do. The important thing is to have some idea where you're going to begin, and that you have a sense of the quality of life you desire.

In chapter 7, we'll take a closer look at goals and help you set some goals for yourself. For now, it's just important that you understand the distinction between values and goals. In the rest of this chapter, we'll help you explore your personal values. As we do so, keep in mind the distinction between values and goals, or you might get stuck. Values are lifelong paths that vitalize your life by giving it direction and meaning. You live your values all your life; they never end. Goals, on the other hand, have an end point.

People often experience many kinds of pain and heartache when they meet their goals. More likely than not, your own life experiences have taught you how it can feel after a goal is achieved. There's a sense of triumph, but also a letdown. Many people face such a letdown after they graduate from school, finish a big project, get married, or have children. One of the reasons is that they mistake their goals for their values. If you use goals as your compass bearing, once you achieve them it feels as though there's nothing left to do in life. For example, if you feel as though the meaning in your life is derived from the goal of graduating from school, what happens when that goal is achieved? Life feels empty.

However, if exploring your intellectual development is something you value and graduating from school is a goal in the service of that value, then when you achieve your goal, there's still more work to do. Values enrich your life with the possibility of constant growth. Goals should be set in the service of that growth and not mistaken for the desire that motivates that growth. This gives us our second important clue about values: They are lifelong paths that contain, but are not bounded by, the things we do in order to live them out.

YOUR VALUES: EXPLORING TEN LIFE DOMAINS

Now that you have a basic understanding of what we mean by values, let's get moving on exploring your values. We'll explore ten different domains in which people develop values (Hayes, Strosahl, and Wilson 1999). It may be that there are more domains than this, and those we present here could certainly be divided up in different ways. But for the purposes of this book, we'll be using the following domains as a forum for learning more about your values: intimate relationships, parenting, family relationships, social relationships, work, leisure, citizenship, personal growth, health, and spirituality.

EXERCISE: EXPLORING YOUR VALUES

In this exercise, we ask you to think about what is essential to you in each of the ten life domains. What do you want to experience in each realm? Describe each domain as you would have it be in the best of all worlds. Don't describe how it is now or what you have come to settle for or expect. We want you to identify your valued direction in each dimension, what you'll always aspire to regardless of your age or the circumstances of your life.

Intimate relationships: Many different relationships could be defined as intimate, but for the purposes of this book we'll define an intimate relationship as the one you have with that special someone who reflects and completes you. If you're married or have a partner, explore your values in terms of that person. If not, you may want to consider what kind of value you place on this type of intimate relationship in general. Describe in just a few words or sentences the quality of your ideal of an intimate relationship. It might help to think about what this intimate relationship would give you that you value.

_____

_____

_____

_____

Parenting: Earlier in the chapter we followed a fairly extensive example of a woman who wanted to be an engaged mother. For this person, parenting would be a domain she particularly values. Consider your relationships with your children or children in general. If you don't have children, think about where being a parent falls in terms of what you want your life to be about. This domain can also be about your relationship with any child. You don't need to be a parent to cultivate a relationship with a child or young person. Describe the quality of your relationship with a child if it were the way you would like it to be.

_____

_____

_____

_____

Family relationships: These are the relationships you have with all the other members of your family, for example, your brothers and sisters or your parents, perhaps even extended family members, such as your grandparents or in-laws. Ideally, what would you have these relationships be like? What qualities would you bring to your interactions with these people? Describe the quality of these relationships as you would like them to be.

_____

_____

_____

_____

Social relationships: This domain actually encompasses a fairly broad range of people. When thinking in terms of social relationships, you may want to consider your closest friends, your colleagues at work, your acquaintances, or even the way you interact with people you don't know very well or whom you meet by chance. Describe the quality of these interactions if they were exactly the way you would want them to be. What would a social network provide for you?

_____

_____

_____

_____

Work: Work is an area of life that often takes a hit when people have chronic pain. Contributing to society by using your special skills, whether that means being in a valued career or volunteering (for example, at the local school), can generate a lot of meaning for most people. What types of important qualities does having a job, salaried or not, provide for you? Have you put a valued occupation, career, or volunteer job on hold because of your pain? Envision your dream job or how you'd like to use your energy and skills productively. What would that look like? Describe the qualities of a job or endeavor that you believe would be perfect for you.

_____

_____

_____

_____

Leisure: The way you spend your leisure time can profoundly affect your quality of life. Think about what this area of your life means to you. This domain is about your own interests. What are the activities, interests, or hobbies that you would love to cultivate and explore if you could? Describe the quality of this part of your life if it were exactly the way you would like it to be.

_____

_____

_____

_____

Citizenship: For some people, contributing to their community in a positive way is of fundamental importance. This could include social activism, volunteering, or some other philanthropic act. What does being a citizen mean to you? Describe how you would generally like to contribute to the society that you live in, in the best of all worlds. What would it mean to you if you were involved with your community the way you would like to be?

_____

_____

_____

_____

Personal growth: This domain could also be called "education" if you take that term in its broadest sense. We don't necessarily mean traditional schooling here, but that's certainly one possible way to explore your personal growth. Artistic or creative endeavors are another form of personal growth. Personal growth is anything that allows you to more deeply explore and develop who you are. Describe the quality of personal growth and learning that you would like to see for yourself right now and throughout your life, regardless of your age or life circumstances.

_____

_____

_____

_____

Health: How important is your physical health to you? What roles do exercise and the way you eat play in your life? Ask yourself these kinds of questions as you explore this area in the space below. Think about how you'd like to take care of your body in terms of exercise, diet, and sleeping under ideal circumstances and describe that here.

_____

_____

_____

_____

Spirituality: By "spirituality," we don't necessarily mean organized religion, though for some people this may play an important role. Think about spirituality broadly and in your own terms—however seems appropriate to you. Describe the role you'd like to see spirituality play in your life and how that would manifest. If you had this in your life, what kind of qualities would it provide for you?

_____

_____

_____

_____

You'll notice that many of these domains have to do with your relationships with other people. Even more affect or are affected by the people in your life. As you go through this work, remember that your values are not about them, your values are about you. And living in accord with your values isn't about what you think you *should* do, it's about doing what will make you feel vital and alive. It's easy to get wrapped up in what you think other people expect from you and live your life based on those expectations. This is not what values are about. Values are the choices *you* make about what you want *your* life to be about. Of course, this may be influenced by many factors, including the people you care about. Nonetheless, this is about your life and the kind of life you want to live. You're not going to find a vital and meaningful life if you make decisions based on what you think other people want of you. When defining your values in the course of the following exercises, keep yourself in mind. If you could live the life you wanted, what would that look like?

ATTENDING YOUR OWN FUNERAL

What would it be like if you could attend your own funeral? Have you ever thought about that? Many people have. Some people even dream about what people at their funeral might say about them after they pass away. This may seem like a strange proposition, but in this section we'll ask you to explore what it might be like to be at your own funeral (Hayes, Strosahl, and Wilson 1999). Though it may feel scary or sad, this is not an exercise in some sort of macabre brooding. It's done in the service of something much more important—your values.

Your values dictate the journey your life will lead you on. Because of this, it can be useful to imagine what it would be like to get to the end of that journey and look back over your lifetime to see what you were all about. How you judge that life when it's over can be more revealing than what you think about your daily struggles with chronic pain. What you imagine people saying about you at your funeral is another clue about what you value. If you could have people remember you exactly as you want to be remembered, how would that be?

To explore some of these issues, take the time to read through the following instructions and then sit back, close your eyes, and visualize your own funeral (Hayes, Strosahl, and Wilson 1999).

EXERCISE: ATTENDING YOUR OWN FUNERAL

Imagine you have died and by some miraculous twist of fate you're able to attend your own funeral in spirit. You float above the ceremony, watching and listening to all that is said and done. You see the procession. You watch the burial or the cremation. Take the time to bring to mind each component of your ideal funeral. Make the scene live in your mind. Where would it be? Would it be at a family burial ground? Perhaps you would have the ceremony by the ocean where you would like your ashes to be scattered. What kind of ceremony would you have? Is it formal or informal? Are there flowers at your funeral?

Now imagine the people you would like to see there commemorating your life. Imagine that anyone living or dead could come to your funeral. Perhaps you see a long-lost friend arriving at the scene. Or perhaps you see a procession of deceased loved ones paying you their respects. This group of people, who have come to remember your life, start giving eulogies about you. Imagine that people associated with each of the first eight domains (save health and spirituality until a bit later) listed above stand up and speak a few words about the kind of person you were. Perhaps your children stand and grieve their loss. Maybe a valued teacher speaks about how dedicated you were to your education. Perhaps your best friend, with whom you loved to vacation, stands and speaks about the trips you took together. What might your spouse or partner say? Who knows, you might even want to imagine what your parents would say. Remember, you can have anyone speak on your behalf at this funeral in your mind.

When you have these people firmly in mind, list them in the spaces provided below. Try to think of at least one person to speak on your behalf in each of the eight domains listed below. If you'd like to list more than one person for any domain, feel free to do that.

Intimate relationships: _____

Parenting: _____

Family relationships: _____

Social relationships: _____

Work: _____

Leisure: _____

Citizenship: _____

Personal growth: _____

Now think about what each of these people is saying about you as you listen to them eulogize you. What qualities do these people remember you for? What did they admire in you? What was it in you that brought them to this funeral? Why do they care about you so much? What did you represent to them? Consider your ideal life and think about how each of these people would remember you if those ideals were met. In the following spaces, make some notes about particular things each of the people in these eight domains recall about you as they remember your life.

Intimate relationships: _____

_____

_____

_____

Parenting: _____

_____

_____

_____

Family relationships: _____

_____

_____

_____

Social relationships: _____

_____

_____

_____

Work: _____

_____

_____

_____

Leisure: _____

_____

_____

_____

Citizenship: _____

_____

_____

_____

Personal growth: _____

_____

_____

_____

Let's take this process a step further. This next part may sound particularly weird to you, but try to stick with it and see where it takes you.

Imagine that by some incredibly strange metaphysical phenomenon there are two more entities in attendance at your funeral—your body and your soul. These two parts of yourself represent the domains of health and spirituality. Imagine your body and soul have the ability to stand up and say a few words about what it was like to be a part of you. Again, assuming you had lived your ideal life, how would your body and soul remember you? What would they say? Take a few moments to make some notes about this in the spaces below.

Your body: _____

_____

_____

_____

Your soul: _____

_____

_____

_____

Once you've completed this exercise, take some time to review your answers. How many of the notes you took revolved around your pain? We're betting that not very many did. When people with chronic pain look at their lives from the perspective offered in this exercise, they're often surprised to find how little of what they want to be remembered for has anything to do with their pain. Generally speaking, people with chronic pain want to be remembered, even by their own body and soul, not as a person who spent a lot of time trying to control chronic pain, but as a loving partner, a good parent, a compassionate friend, a dedicated student, a person who worked for positive change in the world, or a person who delves deeply into the mysteries of life. None of these things are dependent on or diminished by your current struggle with pain. You are free, at this very moment, to pursue any of the things you just wrote about. Your pain does not define you. What does define you are the values by which you live; those things for which you'd like to be remembered. Let's see if we can get a little closer to knowing what those values are.

BUILDING YOUR VALUES COMPASS

The previous exercises in this chapter will have given you some ideas about what your values are. However, we want to help you develop a comprehensive assessment of your values in each of the ten domains. This will include a statement about what your values are, as well as an assessment of how closely you're living in accord with your values right now. This will be your values compass, a set of information that can give your life direction. By the end of this chapter, when you look at your values compass, you should know where you want to go.

EXERCISE: DEVELOPING VALUES STATEMENTS

The first step in creating your values compass is deciding what you want your life to be about. In your ideal world, what would your life be about? Consider this in conjunction with the information you gathered about your values in the previous exercises. Once you've done this, generate a statement that reflects what you want your life to be about in each of the ten domains. Come up with statements that speak to the direction you want to move in during your entire lifetime. The statements should be real in the sense that they genuinely reflect your wishes and intentions, but they shouldn't be ultimately attainable. Remember, these are values, not goals, so they should speak to how you want to live every day of your life but have no end point at which you can say, "Now I've accomplished that."

Throughout this chapter we've given you some ideas about how you might formulate such statements. If you feel stuck, review this chapter and your answers to the previous exercises. You can also refer to Beth's values statements, which appear below, as a guide, but do try to come up with your own ideas before referring to Beth's values statements. It's important that your values come from you. Often our minds hear something that sounds like a good value and we glom onto it, taking it for our own though we may not truly care about it. Really make an effort to come up with statements rooted in your own experience and feelings. The more you do so, the more likely it is that your statements will reflect what you truly value. Describe the quality of each domain as you would have it in the best of all worlds. Imagine that that statement will hold true till your last breath. Here's another way of putting this: If your feet were your values, which way would they go? What types of activities would you engage in to help you move in that direction?

Once you've thought about it, fill in your values statements in the spaces below.

Intimate relationships: _____

_____

Parenting: _____

_____

Family relationships: _____

_____

Social relationships: _____

_____

Work: _____

_____

Leisure: _____

_____

Citizenship: _____

_____

Personal growth: _____

_____

Health: _____

_____

Spirituality: _____

_____

As you'll recall from chapter 1, Beth is an assistant teacher who injured her shoulder and had surgery, but never really recovered from the injury. Eventually she started suffering with chronic pain to such a degree that she nearly lost her job. Just like you, Beth pursued ACT to help her regain her quality of life. To better understand her values, she imagined attending her own funeral just as you did earlier in the chapter. Beth found this a profoundly powerful experience and started crying in her therapist's office. Looking at what she valued through the eyes of the people she cared about revealed the possibility of living a different kind of life than the one she felt she had been relegated to by her pain. She realized that her attempts to control pain had been keeping her from living in accordance with her values. This realization inspired Beth to forge ahead into the work her ACT therapist recommended. Part of this work was developing values statements, just as you did above. Here are the values statements Beth came up with.

BETH'S VALUES STATEMENTS

Intimate relationships: *I want to feel loved and accepted as I am, with my imperfections. I want to give and receive love, physically and spiritually.*

Parenting: *I want to be present for my children when we're together, to show my love and be a good role model.*

Family relationships: *I want to be honest and loving in my relationships with family, expressing my own needs to them rather than just taking care of them.*

Social Relationships: *I want to have friends I can talk to about everything, friends I feel close to and can laugh and cry with.*

Work: *I want to have a job where I can make a contribution and help children, and where I can continue to develop myself.*

Leisure: *I want to spend more time in nature, and I'd love to have space in my life to work with my creative talents, like weaving and painting.*

Citizenship: *I'd like to be one of the people who helps those children in our community who need more caring adult support.*

Personal growth: *I love the feeling of learning new things and want to keep learning for my entire life.*

Health: *I want to feel physically strong and healthy. I want to take care of my body by eating well, getting enough exercise, and getting enough sleep.*

Spirituality: *I want to take time to reflect on life and the harmony that underlies everything. I want to feel like a whole person.*

VALUES ILLNESS

In chapter 2 we gave you a brief overview of values illness, the state people fall into when they let their chronic pain problem take them away from living the life they value. When you sacrifice the life you want to live to control or contain your pain, the vitality is drained from your daily life. Throughout this chapter you've developed a clearer understanding of what you would ideally like your life to be about. If you aren't living that life right now, today, you are suffering from values illness.

This isn't a condemnation, nor should it be a new yardstick by which you consider yourself successful or a failure in life. Such concepts and judgments are part of language-based mental rules we discussed earlier in this chapter in association with relational frame theory. We'll discuss this more later in the book, but for now, suffice it to say that suffering from values illness doesn't mean you are a bad person or a failure.

You may feel sad as you come to realize that you haven't been living the life you truly want to live. Grief is healthy in this sort of context. It's a message that something is wrong. With that knowledge, you can start moving in the direction you truly want to travel.

EXERCISE: COMPLETING YOUR VALUES COMPASS AND ASSESSING THE SEVERITY OF YOUR VALUES ILLNESS

We want to help you determine how severe your values illness is. To accomplish this, you'll fill out your values compass. First, fill in your values statements in the boxes for each of the life domains. You'll note that there are two small blank boxes attached to each value. These boxes are for rating each value in two different ways: in terms of your intentions and in terms of your actions. First, in the top right hand corner, rate how important this value is in your life as a whole. Rate it on a scale of 0 to 10, where 0 means it's not at all important and 10 means it's of the greatest importance to you. Keep in mind that these ratings are not comparative. That is to say, you don't have to judge different values against one another. You could score every single one of them high if you choose to.

Once you've rated how important each value is to you, think about how close you are to manifesting those values in your life today. Are you currently living your values the way you want to? Give this some thought, then rate yourself in the bottom right hand corner on how close you are to carrying out your values in your day-to-day life. Use a rating scale from 0 to 10, 0 meaning you're not living out that value at all and 10 meaning you're living out that value just as you wish to. Once you've finished filling in your ratings in your own values compass, take a look at how Beth rated herself.

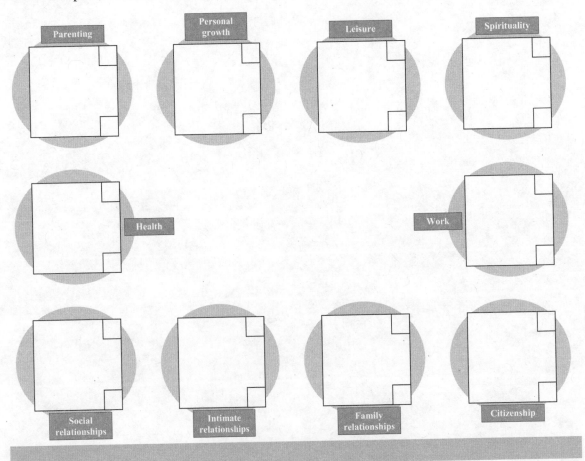

BETH'S VALUES COMPASS

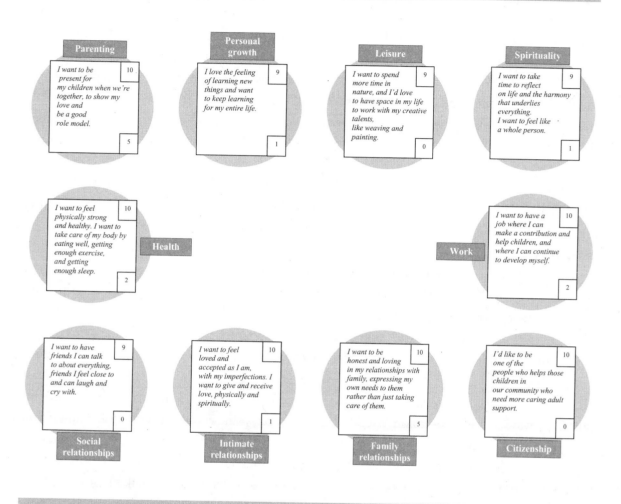

Parenting — 10 / 5
I want to be present for my children when we're together, to show my love and be a good role model.

Personal growth — 9 / 1
I love the feeling of learning new things and want to keep learning for my entire life.

Leisure — 9 / 0
I want to spend more time in nature, and I'd love to have space in my life to work with my creative talents, like weaving and painting.

Spirituality — 9 / 1
I want to take time to reflect on life and the harmony that underlies everything. I want to feel like a whole person.

Health — 10 / 2
I want to feel physically strong and healthy. I want to take care of my body by eating well, getting enough exercise, and getting enough sleep.

Work — 10 / 2
I want to have a job where I can make a contribution and help children, and where I can continue to develop myself.

Social relationships — 9 / 0
I want to have friends I can talk to about everything, friends I feel close to and can laugh and cry with.

Intimate relationships — 10 / 1
I want to feel loved and accepted as I am, with my imperfections. I want to give and receive love, physically and spiritually.

Family relationships — 10 / 5
I want to be honest and loving in my relationships with family, expressing my own needs to them rather than just taking care of them.

Citizenship — 10 / 0
I'd like to be one of the people who helps those children in our community who need more caring adult support.

The greater the discrepancy between how deeply you value a domain and how you're currently manifesting that in your life, the more you suffer from values illness. Again, this isn't something to beat yourself up over. You'll notice that Beth had a bad case of values illness, as many people with chronic pain do. She decided to take the information she gained from exploring her values and use it as inspiration to stick with ACT and learn how to bring her life into alignment with her values. We offer you the same opportunity in this book. If you find that chronic pain has driven you away from the life you truly value and you feel caught in the trap of dirty pain, we can help you find a way out of that maze. If you want to breathe new life into your days, we can help you achieve that goal. That's what ACT for chronic pain is ultimately all about: learning to live the life you want to live rather than being inhibited by your struggles with pain.

WHAT ABOUT THE PAIN?

"But," you may ask, "what about the pain?" You may have noticed that we didn't discuss or explore your pain a great deal. That's because we were investigating what you want your life to be about. We doubt that you want your life to be about a struggle with pain. You are so much more than the pain that has defined much of your recent existence. In this chapter you had the opportunity to find out what some of those things are and remember that you're much bigger than your pain. You want your life to be about more than chronic pain.

Nonetheless, the pain is still there. We don't want to take a Pollyanna attitude about that. We know that you hurt. But consider whether trying to win this battle with pain is really worth all the sacrifices you've made in the service of that objective. Wouldn't it be more fruitful to turn the whole system on its head and live in the service of your values instead? That's the message we hope you'll take from this chapter. We hope it's given you the inspiration to live in the service of what you truly value. That glimmer of hope can drive the work you'll do in the rest of this book.

The following chapters will help you learn to separate yourself from the word games your mind plays with your pain and observe your thoughts, feelings, and actions from a mindful perspective. You'll also learn how to accept your pain (believe it or not) and, ultimately, how to take committed steps toward manifesting the life you want to live in practical ways. The foundation for all this work is your values. Living the values you explored in this chapter is a rewarding alternative to the control trap you've been stuck in for so long. We hope that what you've learned about your values will inspire you to take the next step down a vital, meaningful life path. We hope to help you make this valued life a reality.

CHAPTER 4

Your Thoughts Are Not
What They Say They Are

In the last few chapters we've hinted at something we'll now propose more boldly: You and your thoughts are not the same thing (Hayes, Strosahl, and Wilson 1999). For some of you this may seem like a fairly radical proposal. For others, it may seem self-evident. In any event, we're guessing that right now you identify more with your thinking than you think you do. Because the human mind works on a problem-solution model, we're accustomed to locating problems and then trying to eliminate them. In the outside world this can be a very effective tool. For example, if your car breaks down, you apply your brain to the problem, come up with possible reasons for the breakdown, and then go about solving that problem, perhaps by taking the car to a mechanic, perhaps by repairing the engine yourself. Since this style of thinking is so pervasive and effective in so many scenarios, we humans start to identify ourselves almost completely with our thoughts. We think our thinking dictates who we are and how we need to act. That is, we look *from* our thoughts rather than *at* our thoughts (Hayes, Strosahl, and Wilson 1999).

While incredibly effective in the outside world, when we apply this problem-solution model of thinking and acting to our interior world, particularly to something like chronic pain, we are fighting a losing battle. Chronic pain, by its very definition, is pain that doesn't go away. If you try to solve a problem that's unsolvable, you get stuck in a kind of tug-of-war (Hayes, Strosahl, and Wilson 1999). On one side is your pain, a powerful monster that pulls with all its might on one side of the rope. On the other side is another powerful entity: you and your problem-solving brain, using every bit of your strength to win this battle of will and might. Your chronic pain pulls harder and harder, offering you more and more pain. You pull back using all kinds of different therapies and medications in an attempt to make the pain go away, to beat the monster in this awful game. How long has this tug-of-war been going on? Have you gotten the sense that maybe you can't win this particular battle?

Being caught in this struggle is the essence of what we described in chapter 2 as dirty pain. Not only do you have the physical pain that comes naturally with your condition, you have the additional pain that comes with all the wasted energy, lost opportunities, and life changes you've made in order to try to win this tug-of-war. Go back and review the clean and dirty pain diary you started in chapter 2. How much of your current pain is dirty pain? Noting this will give you a sense of how much you currently identify with your thoughts about pain, and how much energy you've been putting into getting rid of it. The way you think about your pain has drawn you into a battle that you may not ever be able to win. So if you can't win this battle, what alternatives do you have?

You touched on the answer to this question in the previous chapter. One alternative may be to pursue a life you value instead of pursuing a life trying to eliminate your pain. But in order to do this, you will probably have to drop the rope. That is, you'll have to walk away from the tug-of-war you've been engaged in for so long. It is possible. Many people in chronic pain who have been treated with ACT have pursued this path and found great satisfaction in doing so. However, it isn't easy. It's not that it's hard in the traditional sense. Rather, it's tricky. As you may have already noticed, ACT proposes some concepts and skills that may, at first glance, seem counterintuitive or even ridiculous. Nonetheless, as outlined in chapter 1, there's a fair body of research suggesting that the concepts and skills central to ACT are effective and helpful for people in chronic pain.

One of the trickier concepts in the ACT repertoire is the core of this chapter: Your thoughts are not what they say they are (Hayes, Strosahl, and Wilson 1999). For people who are used to identifying themselves with their thoughts (that's most of us!) this idea can be a bit hard to swallow. So this chapter will focus on helping you learn how to develop some distance from your thoughts and look at them for what they are, not what they say they are. This is done in the service of taking you one step closer to living the valued life you explored in the previous chapter, not as some sort of psychological game or philosophical exploration. If you want to start living your valued life, looking at the situation through the lens of your thoughts about pain isn't the most powerful place to be. If you could take a step back and start to look at your thoughts rather than from your thoughts, what would that mean for you?

GETTING DISTANCE FROM YOUR THOUGHTS

In ACT we use the term *cognitive defusion* to describe the act of getting distance from your thoughts (Hayes, Strosahl, and Wilson 1999). "Defusion" is not a word you'll find in any dictionary. It's a word that ACT therapists have come up with to describe a particular psychological event. Looking at the term a little more carefully can help explain why it's important to gain distance from your thoughts.

Most of us operate from a place in which we are fused with our thoughts. We draw little or no distinction between what our mind thinks and how we view ourselves. In the next chapter you'll learn that this is only one way of understanding oneself, and a very limited one at that. Later on, we'll explore other ways of exploring the self; for now, suffice it to say that the totality of who you are is neither dictated nor encompassed by the thoughts you have about your chronic pain condition. It is, however, incredibly easy to get caught in the trap of thinking this is the case. To get a clearer picture of this, fill in the statements below with the first thing that comes to mind.

I am a person who _____

The best thing about me is _____

The worst thing about me is _____

What did you write down? Perhaps you finished the sentence "I am a person who" with the phrase "has chronic pain." How true is this statement? On the one hand, it does identify one aspect of your experience and from this perspective it is a true statement. You are indeed a person who has chronic pain, otherwise you wouldn't be reading this book. But aren't you also a person who has and is and does many other things as well? For example, you might have completed that same sentence with the words "has the ability to breathe." This statement is equally true. In fact you could have completed that same sentence in a million different ways and each of them would be equally true. You are large. You contain multitudes.

In and of itself, there's nothing particularly harmful about a statement like "I am a person who has chronic pain"—as long as it's used as a simple descriptive statement, just as you might say, "I am a person who has the ability to breathe." The problem comes when you fuse your self with particular thoughts. When you buy into a statement like "I am a person who has chronic pain" as a singular truth about you, this simple sentence takes on enormous dimensions. Since you've probably built up a set of rules surrounding your pain over the years, when you fuse with the thought "I am a person who has chronic pain," you call into effect all of those rules. To understand how cognitive fusion has impacted you, specifically, let's take a look at some of the rules you've developed around your pain.

EXERCISE: EXPLORING YOUR RULES ABOUT PAIN

Use the worksheet below to explore some of your own rules about pain. Don't think too hard about it, just write down any rules that pop into your head in the various areas we've suggested. Once you've written down your rules in the left-hand column, write what each rule leads to in the right-hand column. If you need more space, feel free to make additional copies. If you need some help to get you going on this exercise, take a look at the sample worksheet from Beth, which appears below.

Rules	What your rules lead to
1. Rules about pain and work	
2. Rules about feeling pain	
3. Rules about pain and intimate relationships	
4. Rules about pain and justice	
5. Rules about pain and exercise	

BETH'S RULES ABOUT PAIN

Rules	What your rules lead to
1. Rules about pain and work	
I can't work if I'm in pain.	*Once the pain is gone I'll go back to work.*
I can't use any pain medications while on the job.	*Again, fix the pain so I can stop using the medications.*
2. Rules about feeling pain	
Feeling pain is unacceptable. I can't live a good life with that feeling.	*I have to get rid of the pain before I can live a good life.*
It must be a punishment that I'm in this kind of pain, otherwise it would never have happened.	*I'm inherently bad for being in pain and won't be good until I can get out of it.*
3. Rules about pain and intimate relationships	
There's no reason to try to get close to my husband again, because he won't love me while I'm in pain.	*I am unattractive. My husband will leave me and I'll have to learn to live alone.*
4. Rules about pain and justice	
It simply isn't fair that I should suffer with this.	*The world is a cruel and unfair place.*
There are so many bad people in the world and I try to do good, yet still I am punished with this.	*It must be someone else's fault that I'm in so much pain.*
5. Rules about pain and exercise	
Exercising while in pain is not an option.	*I won't exercise until I'm out of pain.*
Exercising will make the pain worse.	*Fix the pain and then start exercising.*

What you've just explored is only a handful of the rules you have likely generated in regard to pain. If you were to try, you could come up with many, many more in relation to all sorts of areas of your life. Some of these rules are absolutely arbitrary, and many have no evidence to support them. Yet for all that, look at how much they cost you in terms of living the valued, engaged life you want to live.

Take a look at how Beth completed this exercise. The rules she's generated over the years as a means of protecting herself from feeling pain have cost her a great deal in terms of living her valued life. How much dirty pain has she caused herself in her attempts to escape the clean pain of her condition? For starters, as a consequence of her rules, Beth believed she wasn't worthy of love, couldn't go back to work, and couldn't exercise. She even believed that she was somehow inherently flawed and was being punished for it. Buying into that led her away from the life she wanted to be living.

Just how much truth is there in any of these rules anyway? While there may be a grain of truth in some of the rules you've created over the years, others are untrue at every level. Either way, the level of truth in any of your rules is not really the issue. What is the issue is how functional your life is. If you buy into a statement like "I am a person who has chronic pain," there's a lot that goes along with the statement. You may not even be fully conscious of what buying into this statement has cost you.

What are the ramifications of being fused with this kind of thought? In the previous chapter you explored your values and rated the level at which you are currently living those values. Looking from your thoughts without being aware of them can cost you the valued life you really want to be living. If your values compass indicated that you aren't currently living in alignment with your values, cognitive fusion may be at least partly responsible for this. At its worst, cognitive fusion puts you in a position where thoughts you don't entirely believe or trust dictate the course of your life.

THE PROBLEM WITH COGNITIVE FUSION—REVISITED

Perhaps the worst part about all this business with cognitive fusion is that it's even more insidious than it looks on the surface. The discussion above reveals only one level of fusion you may have with your thoughts. There is a deeper and more difficult level we need to address before we can move on to the real work of this chapter—cognitive defusion.

As we've mentioned, the mind is a rule maker and a language-based problem-solving machine. It takes in information and immediately goes to work on "solving" it with all the resources of logic at its disposal. Consequently, we humans have a natural tendency that works against us when we receive information such as that presented above, describing rules and fusion. Do you have any idea what that might be? What does your mind tell you when it's convinced itself that rules are bad?

Let's take a look at this. Say, for example, you have a rule that you aren't worthy of love because of your chronic pain. This rule is patently absurd. If you look at it with any objectivity whatsoever, you can logically deduce that this is an unsound concept. As a consequence of this realization, your mind might give you another statement that's seemingly contradictory to the original statement. For example, your mind might tell you, "The idea that you aren't worthy of love because you're in pain is simply not true." This is a seemingly helpful remedy to the original idea that you aren't worthy of love. If you can convince yourself that you *are* worthy of love, perhaps everything will be okay.

Much of our culture, as well as certain schools of psychology, teaches us that this is the reasonable way to respond to unreasonable information. When you realize that a statement like "I'm not worthy of love because I have pain" is an illogical thought that's causing you a great deal of distress, you counter it with an idea like "I'm worthy of love even though I have pain." The problem here is quite tricky. Contained in the statement "I am worthy of love even though I have pain" is an implicit reference to the idea that you are, in fact, *not* worthy of love. Think about it: If you're busy countering thoughts that come up in regard to a rule like this, don't you have to think of the rule first in order to counter it? So here you are again, stuck to the rule you're trying to get rid of.

In exploring your rules above, you may have been tempted to counter them with seemingly more logical rules, or you may have simply denied they were true in the first place. If you found yourself doing either, you're getting caught in one of the most elegant and dangerous traps your mind can set for you. Don't judge yourself harshly for this; it's simply something to be aware of as you move forward with the defusion exercises in this chapter. Defusion is not a means to fight against your thoughts or deny their existence.

There's another trick your mind can play that you should be aware of as we move forward. In the face of thoughts like "I am a person who has chronic pain" or any of the rules you've generated surrounding this statement, your mind might offer you the solution of simply not thinking about it. This is something people with chronic pain tend to do quite a lot, and it manifests in a number of different ways. Because the pain is so pervasive, and because you so badly want to be rid of it, you'll be tempted to try to put it out of your mind. You may find yourself doing the same thing with negative thoughts that surround the pain. When you run into rules like "I'm not worthy of love because I have pain," you may be tempted to simply push the thought away. It turns out this is as dangerous as trying to fight with the thought. The reason goes back to experiential avoidance, which we discussed in chapter 1. Avoiding thoughts by trying to push them out of your mind is simply another type of experiential avoidance.

Just as with trying to counter negative thoughts with positive ones, trying to avoid a thought actually brings that thought to mind (Hayes, Strosahl, and Wilson 1999). Try the following exercise to experiment with how this works.

EXERCISE: DON'T THINK OF CHOCOLATE ICE CREAM

Here's an unusual request: For the next few minutes, do *not* think of chocolate ice cream. Whatever you do, try not to think of any of your experiences with chocolate ice cream. Don't think about the creamy texture or the delicious taste of chocolate. Don't think of it in an ice cream cone, dripping over the side and down your fingers. Don't think about how cool and refreshing it is on a warm day. Don't think of your favorite experiences taking your children, friends, or family out for ice cream. Don't think about having fun eating ice cream when you were a kid. Under no circumstance are you to think about chocolate ice cream. Think of anything else but chocolate ice cream.

Take a few minutes and really put some effort into not thinking about chocolate ice cream. Start now.

What did you think about during those few minutes? _____

_____

_____

_____

Let's imagine for a moment that you were successful in not thinking of chocolate ice cream and that you wrote something else in the space above. How do you know you weren't thinking of chocolate ice cream? You have to bring the thought of chocolate ice cream to mind to know that you "weren't" thinking about it. To intentionally not think about something calls that very thing to mind, whether it be chocolate ice cream or thoughts about pain.

This is why experiential avoidance doesn't work; it simply can't. Each attempt you make to eliminate an experience calls to mind that very experience along with everything associated with it. If you try to push something out of your mind, you're paradoxically left with that very thing. In ACT we use the phrase "If you don't want it, you've got it" to describe this state. What this suggests in terms of cognitive fusion is that attempts to fight thoughts with thoughts or avoid them entirely are still fused ways of interacting with your thinking. If you don't want it, you've got it; if you don't want to think it, you've thought it. The solutions our mind gives us as alternatives to cognitive fusion are themselves fused ways of operating.

WHY DEFUSION?

In this chapter, we present an alternative to cognitive fusion: cognitive defusion (Hayes, Strosahl, and Wilson 1999). If being fused with your thoughts is the point at which you are looking from your thoughts rather than at them, defusion is the point at which you are looking at your thoughts rather than from them. Defusion is the ability to watch your thoughts come and go without attaching yourself to them. Defusion allows you to have thoughts without putting those thoughts in the driver's seat of your life. This is a skill you can acquire, and in the remainder of this chapter we'll help you learn how to do it.

You may be wondering why to bother with defusion. One thing is certain, defusion isn't going to solve your pain problem the way you might hope it will. It won't make your pain go away, and it won't make your thoughts about the pain go away. In fact, if you hope defusion will be a panacea, erasing your pain, then you're trying to use defusion as a means of experiential avoidance and hence are still acting from a fused state! As we said, these concepts are tricky. If this isn't completely clear to you, reread the section above on experiential avoidance.

What defusion can offer you is the means to gain enough distance from your thoughts to make choices on your own, without the influence of the ever-buzzing mind machine at your back. Once you learn to notice your thoughts and look *at* them instead of *from* them, you can bring your entire self to bear on making choices about your life (Hayes, Strosahl, and Wilson 1999). You may remember from the previous chapter that values are all about choices. Learning to defuse from your thoughts can help put you in a position to choose the valued life you've been missing while you were steeped in your struggle with pain. Defusion helps you drop the rope in your tug-of-war with pain and move on with a vital life that you can cherish.

Again, please remember that the exercises in this chapter are not another yardstick by which you should judge your success or failure as a human being. You are not meant to be perfectly and eternally defused from your thinking. In fact, you wouldn't want to be. Sometimes fusing with your thoughts is a very valuable tool. When you're repairing your car or completing your income tax return, there's little to be gained by defusing from your thoughts; it might even be counterproductive. In truth, it's simply inefficient in those contexts. What these exercises are meant to do is expand your repertoire of psychological responses, hence increasing your psychological flexibility. And increasing psychological flexibility has been shown to have profoundly positive impacts for people who suffer from chronic pain (Dahl, Wilson, and Nilsson 2004).

As with all the material presented in this book, we encourage you to work on cognitive defusion so that you can live a fuller, more engaged, more vital, more workable life. Defusion won't heal your physical pain, but it might help heal your suffering and repair the broken parts of your life.

Painful Thinking

As you start to work on defusion, it's useful to figure out how much of the time you're preoccupied with thoughts about your pain. Beyond that, finding out exactly what those thoughts are, when they tend to come up, and what kinds of actions they lead to will give you a practical basis for your work in defusion. Therefore, before we get started on the actual defusion exercises, we ask that you take some time to document what we'll call your "painful thinking." Various exercises in previous chapters may have given you some ideas about painful thoughts you may be having. Let's zero in on this aspect of your experience with pain a little more closely.

EXERCISE: PAINFUL THINKING DIARY

For the next week, focus in on any thoughts related to your pain. To this end, make seven photocopies of the following worksheet and keep it with you at all times. Each time a thought pops up about your pain, note it in the appropriate space. Although the worksheet is divided up into hourly segments, if you have more than one thought about pain in an hour, feel free to note multiple thoughts. If there's not enough space on this worksheet to record all of your pain-related thoughts, you can use a notebook or journal. When you find yourself in a situation where it's inconvenient to make such notes (for example, in the supermarket or when giving a presentation), write down your experience as soon as you can. Some of the spaces on the sheet may stay blank (for example, 2 A.M.). Again, this isn't a problem. But if you wake up in the middle of the night with thoughts about your pain, do write them down. There's no right or wrong way to fill in this thought diary. Its primary purpose is to give you an idea how much "painful thinking" you currently engage in.

In addition to taking notes on the content of each painful thought, rank the intensity of each thought on a scale from 1 to 10, 10 being the most intense. Also note what actions, if any, the thought leads to. For example, if the thought "This pain has destroyed my life" comes up and it's very strong, you might rank the intensity of that thought at 10. If the thought makes you want to have a drink or pop a pain pill, note that in the right-hand column. Following the blank worksheet, we've provided an example from Beth's painful thinking diary.

Once you've recorded your painful thoughts for an entire week, come back to the book and finish working on the chapter.

PAINFUL THINKING DIARY

Time	Thought about pain	Intensity	Actions the thought leads to
12 A.M.			
1 A.M.			
2 A.M.			
3 A.M.			
4 A.M.			
5 A.M.			
6 A.M.			
7 A.M.			
8 A.M.			
9 A.M.			
10 A.M.			
11 A.M.			
12 P.M.			
1 P.M.			
2 P.M.			
3 P.M.			
4 P.M.			
5 P.M.			
6 P.M.			
7 P.M.			
8 P.M.			
9 P.M.			
10 P.M.			
11 P.M.			

BETH'S PAINFUL THINKING DIARY

Time	Thought about pain	Intensity	Actions the thought leads to
12 A.M.			
1 A.M.			
2 A.M.			
3 A.M.			
4 A.M.			
5 A.M.			
6 A.M.	Woke up with that same shoulder pain. I can't go through my day like this.	7	Took a pain pill to relieve the pain.
7 A.M.	Sat down to breakfast. I can't even pick up a spoon without thinking of the pain.	5	Wanted to throw out my breakfast.
8 A.M.	I would be going to work right now if it weren't for the pain.	9	Sat down on the couch and cried.
9 A.M.	Stuck here on the sofa watching stupid game shows because of this damned pain.	6	Thought about taking a drink but it seemed too early.
10 A.M.	Was going to get up and go for a walk, but couldn't because I hurt.	6	Went and sat down again.
11 A.M.	I am so alone.	10	Cried some more.
12 P.M.	Wanted to go to lunch with a friend. Thought I shouldn't because of pain.	9	Ate some ramen alone.
1 P.M.	What has my life come to?	10	Took a drink to stop this thought.
2 P.M.			
3 P.M.			
4 P.M.	Normally I'd go watch my son play hockey right now, but I can't because of the pain.	8	Tried to do some stretching, but got fed up and laid down.
5 P.M.	It took all my energy to make dinner, so I couldn't sit with the kids and eat, which led to thinking what a lousy mother I am.	9	Took some pills and went to bed.
6 P.M.	I guess I should just give up.	10	Stared at the ceiling and tried not to feel anything.
7 P.M.	Feel lonely, worthless, and depressed. I wish I could escape the pain.	8	Took another pill and went to bed early.
8 P.M.			
9 P.M.			
10 P.M.			
11 P.M.			

If you're like most people who complete this pain diary, you'll find that your thoughts surrounding pain are more pervasive than you would have imagined. You may even have found it difficult to track them all because there were so many. Sometimes you may have found it difficult to divide the thoughts you had about your pain from other kinds of thoughts. Chronic pain is so deep that it sometimes seems to infiltrate every part of a person's life. None of this means that you're bad or that your thinking is flawed. It's absolutely natural to be having all of these thoughts in the face of such extreme circumstances.

What you should bring away from this exercise is a fairly good understanding of how much of your life is dominated by fusing with thoughts about pain and what that is costing you. Though it could seem disheartening, this is actually a great place to be. Armed with this information, you can choose to react in new ways. Each of your thoughts around your pain presents an opportunity to apply the defusion skills we'll teach you now.

Acquiring the Skills

The following exercises will help you develop the cognitive defusion skills that ACT therapists use to help treat their clients with chronic pain. Each skill is effective in its own right, and each can be used at any time. All of them are equally powerful, and each can help you gain some distance from your thoughts.

The following exercises are presented one after another to make it easier for you to refer to them when you need them. As you forge ahead into this series of exercises, keep a couple of things in mind. First, the information and exercises in this book will be of very limited use if you don't apply them in practical ways in your everyday life. Though you'll begin practicing the following skills in the context of the book, the goal is for you to apply defusion skills in your daily life. Simply reading the text and not making use of it won't get you very far.

Second, there are a lot of cognitive defusion exercises in the ACT literature, and more are being created every day. All of these exercises are built on a set of fundamental principles. Once you have an understanding of the basic concepts at the heart of defusion, you can make up your own techniques if you wish. Ultimately, anything you do to create some distance between you and your thoughts can be called a defusion technique. And the point is not to ameliorate the pain your thoughts cause you, but simply to look at those thoughts a little more objectively. We have found the following set of exercises to be particularly helpful for people with chronic pain, but they are by no means the whole picture. They are but a handful of the techniques that exist for this kind of work.

EXERCISE: THE ARROGANCE OF WORDS

We've talked about how buying into certain ideas can generate a vast array of negative psychological content. This exercise examines just how arrogant words can be, and how they are often only so much wind (Hayes, Strosahl, and Wilson 1999).

In the space below, write down the part of your body that causes you the most pain. Try to make this a short and concise phrase, such as "my back."

_____

Now take a few minutes to write down all of the thoughts and feelings that come up when you speak this phrase aloud or bring it to mind. When you say "my back," what comes up for you?

_____

_____

_____

_____

Once you've done this, find a quiet space where you can be alone and say the phrase you wrote down aloud about one hundred times in a row without stopping. Just keep saying "my back" or whatever else you wrote down over and over again. Do this now.

When you say the words again and again, what happens to them? Do they still have the same effect on you as they did before? Do they bring up all the same psychological content while you're repeating them over and over?

If you are like most people, the words will become slightly disassociated with the negative content they initially produced. In fact, most people who do this exercise end up feeling that the words sound odd or unfamiliar, or that they have no inherent meaning whatsoever. That's because they don't. Words are simply vocalizations we humans make. The meaning we attach to them is not inherent in the sounds themselves any more than it is inherent in the markings you are reading on this page right now. You're the one generating the meaning as you read or speak or think. The words "my back" can be loaded with associations. In the case of someone with chronic back pain, many of those associations are negative. But the words themselves hold no meaning whatsoever. They are just words. Like schoolyard bullies, when confronted with their impotence they tend to deflate. Divorcing the vocalizations from the meanings they usually associate with can alter your perspective in some powerful ways.

EXERCISE: THE THOUGHT OBSERVER

For this exercise, find a street that's fairly busy with traffic. Watch the cars go by and simply name them as they cross your line of vision. You can simply say, "There's a Plymouth; there's a Ford; there's a sedan; there's a station wagon," and so on. Whatever identification system works for you is fine. How long are you able to do this without thinking about anything but the passing cars? Go out and do this and time yourself. Write down your time here:

_____

Thinking is incredibly insidious. The mental word machine that we all have produces thought almost all the time. If you're like most of us, you can only go a very short time simply watching and naming the cars without thinking of anything else. As you watch the cars pass, many different thoughts are likely to come up. Perhaps you see a red Maserati and think "Man, that's an unusual car. I wish I had one." Or perhaps you see a Ford pickup and think "I wish I had a pickup so I could move that stuff in the backyard to the dump. But hell, I might feel that pain in my hip if I started doing that anyway." If you watch carefully, you'll notice that your mind comes up with all kinds of wonderful and bizarre little thoughts as you do an activity like this.

Let's take this exercise one step further. For the next few minutes, write down all the thoughts that come into your mind. You needn't concentrate on anything in particular. Just write down whatever your mind machine comes up with.

_____

_____

_____

_____

You probably found a million and one things coming up during those short few minutes, some related to your pain, some not. Now bring the street where you watched the passing cars to your mind's eye. Imagine that as you have a thought, you can simply attach it to one of the cars and watch it glide past. For example, let's say you had the thought "I hate this stupid pain." Mentally paint those words on the side of a car and watch it disappear down the street with the words attached. Watch your thoughts come up, and watch them simply roll away down the street. Go ahead and do this with the thoughts that are coming up right now. If you're thinking "Wow, this is a really lame exercise," go ahead and put that on the side of a car and watch it go by. On the other hand, if you're thinking "This is really cool and I'm really good at it," put that on the side of a car and watch it go by as well. Do this for a few minutes and watch your mind.

While watching your mind, see if you can find the point when you stop watching the thoughts go by on cars and start looking through the lens of the thoughts themselves. This is the point at which you're sinking into the content generated by your mind, and it happens all the time. Do you find yourself praising or criticizing yourself on your performance in this exercise? If so, you've fallen into a very common mental trap. Any attempt to judge your performance is only your mind generating more thoughts. Do you find yourself becoming caught up in thoughts about pain? Again, this is a common trap. If this is the case, don't be hard on yourself. Rather, try to take those thoughts, paint them on cars, and watch them disappear down the street. This and similar exercises for observing your thoughts can be an incredibly powerful cognitive defusion tool.

EXERCISE: THIS IS ME THINKING . . .

One of the most potentially destructive ways thoughts manifest themselves is as statements about reality. For example, the thought "I am in pain" can identify you and your pain as the same thing. How often does that statement get translated into "I am pain" in your mind? Once this happens, you identify yourself completely with something that's only a small part of your total identity and experience as a human being. Yes, we said "small." Pain may have a big impact on your life, but in the big picture of your life, how much of your daily experience is pain? Aren't there many other things going on as well?

One way you can gain some distance from this kind of thinking is to label the thoughts as thoughts. For example, when you think "I am in pain," it's actually more accurate to state "This is me thinking I am in pain." Don't get us wrong; we're not suggesting that your pain isn't there and isn't real. However, once you come to the mental spot where your mind generates a statement about the pain, even one as simple as "I am in pain," you've started to think about it. And while thinking about your pain isn't in itself bad, it can be very helpful to learn how to separate yourself from those thoughts (Hayes, Strosahl, and Wilson 1999).

Now take a look at your painful thinking diary and find a few recurring thoughts. These can be thoughts that are particularly difficult to cope with or ones that are easier for you to face. For the purposes of this exercise it doesn't matter. Write down the recurring thoughts in the spaces below.

_____

_____

_____

_____

_____

_____

_____

Next, consider how you could more accurately describe what is really going on when these thoughts come to mind, then write these more accurate phrases in the space below. You will find it helpful to use phrases like "This is me thinking . . . ," "I'm having the thought that . . . ," or simply "Thinking . . ." as a prelude to the various statements (Hayes, Strosahl, and Wilson 1999).

_____

_____

_____

_____

_____

_____

_____

_____

Now call each of the thoughts to mind in its new form. How has rephrasing them affected their power over you?

EXERCISE: KICK YOUR BUTS

In this exercise, we'll teach you how to kick some "buts" (Hayes, Strosahl, and Wilson 1999). When we use the word "but," we usually intend to indicate opposition to a statement. For example, you might say "I would love to go to the movies with you tonight, but I am in so much pain." In this case, the word "but" connotes that there's no practical way for you to go to the movies because of your pain.

For the next couple of days, track your "but" thoughts and statements and list them below. If you watch your thoughts carefully, you'll find the word "but" in places you wouldn't necessarily expect it to be. If you're having a hard time finding any "but" thoughts, look through your painful thinking diary to see if you've recorded any there. You might also think about this in terms of the values you explored in chapter 3. What are some directions you might like to take, and what is holding you back? When you think in these terms, are the thoughts formulated as "but" statements in your mind? However you manage it, track your "but" thinking below.

_____ but _____

_____ but _____

_____ but _____

_____ but _____

_____ but _____

_____ but _____

_____ but _____

_____ but _____

Now let's see what happens when you simply replace the word "but" with "and." As an experiment, rewrite your "but" statements as "and" statements in the section below.

_____ and _____

_____ and _____

_____ and _____

_____ and _____

_____ and _____

_____ and _____

_____ and _____

_____ and _____

_____ and _____

What did this do to your "but" statements? How did this affect their meaning? Could it be possible that these "and" statements are as believable as the "but" statements you started with? If this were true—if these new "and" statements are equally as true or valid as your original "but" statements—what would that mean for you in your life?

Let's look at the example we started with in this exercise: "I would love to go to the movies with you tonight, but I am in so much pain." Changing this sentence to an "and" statement would make it read as follows: "I would love to go to the movies with you tonight, and I am in so much pain." This alters the meaning of the original statement in some pretty radical ways. In the first sentence, the word "but" implied that the pain prevented the person from going to the movies. A simple word implied the actions that person can and cannot take. Changing that "but" to "and" suggests something completely different. Using the word "and" in the context of the sentence above suggests that the person can in fact go to the movies *and* still be in pain.

Now reconsider the question we asked above: If you could accept the validity of such "and" statements, how would that alter your life? Take a few moments and jot down some thoughts on this.

This exercise actually contains two separate, related lessons. The first is that you can dramatically alter the course of your life by making simple shifts in your perspective. Changing "but" statements to "and" statements is evidence of this. More importantly, it once again reveals how words have the power to take over your life, and how they affect your actions. If you can change the whole sense of a sentence, even change an idea's practical implications for your life, by altering a single word in that sentence, how much power might words really have over your life?

BEING THE WATCHER

Take these exercises with you into your everyday life. This will increase their potency and expand your awareness of both the prevalence of your pain-related thoughts and the impacts those thoughts currently have on your actions.

Learning that you and your thinking are not the same thing can have a profound influence on your life (Hayes, Strosahl, and Wilson 1999). It can also raise some serious existential questions. You may have gotten a sense of these questions as you worked through the exercises in this chapter. In some cases these questions can be painful and frightening. You may ask yourself, "If I am not my thoughts, who am I?" as a client in ACT therapy once did. For now, simply thank your mind for such thoughts and use the techniques in this chapter to gain a little distance from them. Perhaps that, in itself, will give you some perspective. In any event, we will be addressing these issues in the next chapter on mindfulness.

CHAPTER 5

Mindfulness: The Answer When Your Mind Isn't

In the previous chapter, you were able to get a sense of what it's like to defuse from your thoughts. You may have felt empowered and refreshed by the possibility that you can look at your experience with pain in ways you weren't previously aware of. Cognitive defusion is not an escape mechanism. It isn't a means to get away from the pain, but it is a powerful way to reconceptualize the possibilities that surround your experience with pain. You may now start to see that there are new avenues open to you that you hadn't previously considered. Broadening your repertoire of psychological responses is an important and valuable aspect of the work you're doing in this book. And it has been proven to have many positive effects on people who suffer from chronic pain (McCracken and Eccleston 2003).

But taking distance from your thoughts and learning to look at them rather than from them can be scary. Most of us identify so completely with what we're thinking that getting a sense that there's a difference between one's self and one's thoughts can be a bit unsettling. This experience can raise some difficult existential questions. What does it mean if what you think doesn't define who you are? If your painful thoughts don't define you, doesn't that also imply that your positive thoughts don't truly define you either? If you are not your thoughts, who are you?

For many people who suffer from chronic pain, these questions roll right into the way they identify with the pain itself. One of the sad and difficult aspects of living with chronic pain is that you begin to bind your identity with your pain experience. You start to see yourself as the pain and only the pain rather than as a person who feels pain but also feels many other things. You may even be holding on to your pain as a way to define who you are. Perhaps the pain has been with you so long that you worry you wouldn't even know who you are without pain. The question may then manifest itself as, If you are not your pain, who are you?

In this chapter we'll help provide you some perspective on these questions and perhaps open your eyes to an aspect of yourself that you may not have considered up to this point—the observer self (Hayes, Strosahl, and Wilson 1999). Once you can start to look at your experience, all of your experience, in the larger context of who you truly are, it becomes easier and easier to defuse from your thoughts. This defused awareness of your self as an ongoing process is how we define mindfulness.

Mindfulness is an elder cousin of defusion. This age-old technique has been practiced in Eastern cultures for millennia. Recently it has found its way into the Western psychological sciences, and it's been shown to have incredibly positive effects on people who suffer with any type of mental or physical pain (Dahl, Wilson, and Nilsson 2004). In this chapter, we'll teach you what mindfulness is and how you can apply it daily to your problems with pain. But before we get to that, we need to broaden your understanding of your self. Let's start by investigating the three aspects of self that ACT recognizes.

THE THREE ASPECTS OF SELF

ACT identifies not one but three ways that you can conceive of your self (Hayes, Strosahl, and Wilson 1999). Indeed, there may be others, but for our purposes we'll stick to three. We'll look at each of these ways of understanding your own identity and experience in some detail.

Be aware that examining the different ways you can observe your own experience is not an academic exercise. It's a valuable tool that will allow you to see that your self may be somewhere and something you don't expect it to be. It will help you recognize that there's a place where you can sit, defused from your thoughts, and still have a firm grip on who you are. In fact, you may get a firmer grip on it than you've ever had before.

The three aspects of self that ACT recognizes are the *conceptualized self*, the *self as ongoing awareness*, and the *observer self* (Hayes, Strosahl, and Wilson 1999). Our goal in this chapter is to help you defuse more from your conceptualized self and identify more with your observer self. Let's look at each of these aspects of self in detail.

The Conceptualized Self

The conceptualized self is the mentally defined concept you have of who you are (Hayes, Strosahl, and Wilson 1999). It's you looking at yourself through the lens of your thoughts. It's your mind machine's message to you about who and what you are. This aspect of self incorporates all of your history and your judgments on that history and develops them into a cogent and consistent story that reflects your "self." It is all the ways that you attach your identity to specific concepts or intellectual formulations about who you are. This is the aspect of your self that you're probably most familiar with. It's also the form of your self that you brought into this book with you. This is the self that's most threatened by defusion, because it's most directly tied to your thoughts.

This is the self that has equated you with your pain for so long. Remember the exercise you did in the beginning of chapter 4 where we asked you to complete statements like "I am a person who . . ."? Any answer you gave to any of those statements reflected your conceptualized self. If you filled in the blank to create a statement along the lines of "I am a person who has chronic pain," your conceptualized self was at work in providing that answer.

Let's take that exercise a step further. In the space below, complete the following sentence with every single possibility that comes to mind. (If you really apply yourself, you may need a separate sheet of paper to complete this exercise!)

I am a person who . . .

_____

_____

_____

_____

_____

_____

_____

_____

_____

_____

How many answers did you come up with? How many different ways can you conceive of your self? And yet, which of these really defines you as a complete and total person? Doesn't each of these answers only speak to one aspect of your experience?

Another exercise may help you catch your conceptualized self in motion. Read the following statement and then take notes on everything your mind produces in relation to this statement: I am a perfect and competent individual and have everything I need in order to realize the dreams I want for my life.

_____

_____

_____

_____

_____

_____

_____

_____

Now try the same exercise again with this statement: I am a totally imperfect and incompetent individual and have nothing I need to realize my dreams.

_____

_____

_____

_____

_____

_____

_____

_____

_____

_____

Which of your responses is "true"? Which are real reflections of who you are and what you're capable of? You could probably come up with even more conceptualizations if you wanted to. And which of these would be an accurate representation of your total self?

Human minds are great at coming up with rationalizations for any statement. In fact, at this very moment you might be trying to buy into one of the answers that you gave above. Or you might be ashamed to realize that you weren't able to come up with a "right" answer. Either way, it's just more information from the conceptualized self. You can simply thank your mind for those thoughts and move on with your reading.

Don't get us wrong. The conceptualized self is not inherently bad. It has its uses. You need to identify yourself with particular roles in particular circumstances; otherwise it becomes very difficult to act at all. Imagine that you're a schoolteacher, like Beth, but that you completely abnegate your conceptualized self. How would you know that you were a schoolteacher?

We aren't asking you to get rid of the ways you conceptualize your experience. They are valuable in certain ways. But we want you to see that your experience as a human being isn't limited by what you think about yourself. You are a person who has pain. This is true and cannot be false. But you are also a person who has and is and does many other things. Each of these conceptualizations is part of who you are, but they don't define you. In fact, they're ultimately only tiny, fleeting, ever-changeable aspects of who you are. You are bigger than these concepts you have of yourself.

The Self as Ongoing Awareness

Each of us has a sense of our personal history. Because time moves in one direction and because we are aware of our own existence, we keep a record of who we are in our minds at all times. This isn't inherently good or bad (unless you judge it as such, in which case you've fallen into the world of the conceptualized self). Having the ability to record your own history and remember your own past is valuable. In the social arenas we all live in, this is a very important tool. You would be considered strange if, for example, you couldn't remember what happened in your childhood.

Though your memories don't define who you are, it can be useful to have a record of your history. Imagine you're talking with an old friend and recalling an event that you experienced together when you were kids. You can engage with your friend and chat with him or her about this particular issue because you both have the same memory. If you were to lose that ability, it would make the situation awkward and difficult.

In a similar way, you know the history of your experience with pain. That history includes objective facts that you can share with friends, family members, or medical professionals. These facts can be valuable information as long as you look at them as information. For example, knowing when you first felt the pain that's been crippling your life is a part of your history, and denying that it happened isn't going to do you any good at all.

ACT neither encourages nor discourages your sense of ongoing self-awareness. Rather, it views this aspect of self as a by-product of your ability with language and little more. It can be a fairly neutral manifestation of self as long as you allow it to remain that way.

Problems with ongoing self-awareness crop up when people start judging certain aspects of their history. For example, you may remember the first day you felt pain as the worst day of your life. While that's an understandable conceptualization of the event, it is just that—a conceptualization. It isn't any more real than if you were to think that the first day you felt pain was the best day of your life. Both ways of conceptualizing the experience are based on information that your mind gives you, and neither would be an accurate reflection of historical fact.

That being said, we're not going to devote much more attention to this aspect of self from here on out. Because ACT sees ongoing self-awareness as a neutral event, we won't focus on it very much in this book. We've offered this explanation as a way to prepare you for learning the third aspect of self: the observer self. We'll focus on the observer self for the rest of this chapter.

The Observer Self

There is a self that has always been with you and will always be (Hayes, Strosahl, and Wilson 1999). If you look back over your history, you can easily remember much of what's happened in your life. But you can take this a step further. You can remember what it was like to be there in any given moment. You have the memory of what it was like to be you in the story of your own life as far back as you can remember. *You* were there. But if you are your current conceptualized self, how can you have been there then? Which self are you?

Try the following exercise (Hayes, Strosahl, and Wilson 1999) to see if you can work this riddle out for yourself.

EXERCISE: LOCATING THE OBSERVER SELF

Think of a situation that happened last summer that meant something special to you. Write it down here:

_____

_____

_____

_____

Think of something that happened when you were a teenager that was very special for you. Describe that situation here:

_____

_____

_____

_____

Finally, think of something that happened when you were very young that was special to you and that you remember well. Describe it here:

_____

_____

_____

_____

Now answer this question: Where were *you* in each of these experiences?

_____

_____

_____

_____

Think about you as the self that just observed and described all three of these situations. As you describe what happened to you "then," you're taking on a perspective or creating a space where you observe yourself in a certain context. You observe what happened to you in each of these situations. You are the you watching yourself experiencing what you are experiencing. You are the you who watched each of those special memories from your past happen in real time while you were there. You are also the you in the present moment who remembers those events. You are the you who reads this sentence. You are the you who witnesses everything you experience.

There is an essential connection between the person you are today, the person you were last summer, the person you were as a teenager, and the person you were as a young child. You can probably sense that it's your being behind those observing eyes. This observer self is the stable, unchanging part of yourself. This self sees your self-conceptualizations but is not bound by them; it encompasses each of them. It is you watching yourself as you conceive each of them. The observer self is boundless in the sense that you cannot think or be anything or anywhere outside of it. It is timeless because it has always been with you and will always be with you. Because it cannot be separated from you, it is the most complete representation of who you are. These things are all true for one simple reason: Wherever you go, there you are.

Knowing this makes it less threatening to enter into painful situations, because no matter what happens, you are always going to be observing you; you are always going to be there. No matter how bad things get, no matter how bad the pain is, this observing self will not be threatened or at risk. Your observing self is safe from harm and it will always be there for you because it is you.

Learning how to consciously step into the position of the observer self is a way for you to defuse from your thoughts so you can make choices that come from all of you and move in directions that you value and that give you vitality. Learning how to operate from this perspective is critical to your work with acceptance and mindfulness. When you learn how to do so, it will empower you to live beyond your pain. It will allow you to exist in a space where building the life you've always dreamed of is possible, not in spite of your pain, not after healing from your pain, but right now in this moment with or without whatever pain you are feeling. Let's start working on how you can learn to operate from the perspective of your observer self.

THE CHESSBOARD METAPHOR: LEARNING WHAT MINDFULNESS MEANS

Imagine for a moment that your life is a chess game (Hayes, Strosahl, and Wilson 1999). Each of the pieces on the board represents different ways your mind processes your life situations, conditions, bodily sensations, feelings, or other aspects of your life. Each chess piece has its own characteristic way of operating. You probably know the strategies and patterns of each of your chess pieces because your patterns of struggle have most likely been with you for quite some time now.

These different pieces of your life tend to do the same thing time and again. They divide into teams and start a war inside you. You know the game, it's been going on as long as you can remember. The white pieces and the black pieces fight against one another. On one side, you have "bad" thoughts or feelings, like worrying about your pain, fearing your pain, being depressed by your pain, being anxious about your pain, or feeling uncertain about your life because of your pain; these all hang out together on one side of the board and play for the black team. On the other side, you have your "good" thoughts or feelings, like thinking positively, feeling confident, hoping you can deal with this pain somehow, wishing to have your life back, or feeling momentary happiness from time to time; all these feelings hang out together and play on the other side of the board for the white team. The object of the game is for one of the teams to beat the other; for you to come to some final conclusion about how you're going to deal with your life and the situations your life presents to you.

The battles go on and on, day after day. Some days it looks like the white team is about to win, and some days it looks like the black team will take the victory. Each moment in this endless chess game is about winning or losing battles, no matter how big or small, important or unimportant, they may be. The struggle, which consists of challenging positions, protecting territory, gaining advantages, and finally checkmating the opponent's king, goes on constantly whether you like it or not. Sometimes these battles are over important issues, like the pros and cons of making an important move in life, and sometimes they're about things that are not at all important, like what to wear on a given day. Some days they revolve around your struggle with pain; some days they don't. But they never cease. The pieces just keeping battling on and on. They seem never to tire or be defeated. They play for an eternity.

The Battle Between Living a Valued Life and Protecting Yourself from Pain

Let's take this metaphor a step further. Imagine that one of the battles frequently played out right now in your life is between your valued life and efforts to protect yourself from pain. On the white side are all your dreams and visions of the valued life you most want to live. On the black side are all the thoughts, rules, and ideas your mind has produced regarding how you are to prevent, avoid, or escape your pain.

Your pain plays the position of the king on the black team. All the other players on the black team are saddled with the responsibility of protecting this king from further exposure or injury. They try to protect you by looking for reasons to stop you from taking steps in directions that may end up causing you pain. The white team's king is your valued life. The job of the players on the white team is to protect that king—to try to aid you in taking steps in your valued direction and keep you from losing sight of what is most important to you. The individual chess pieces on the white team are each fighting for a different dimension of your valued life. They're fighting for your self-actualization in each of the areas we discussed in chapter 3: intimate relationships, parenting, family relationships, social relationships, work, leisure, citizenship, personal growth, health, and spirituality.

Here are a few examples of the moves and countermoves each side makes in this battle between the life you value and your attempts to avoid pain.

Valued action: I want to learn and develop as a person. I want to move toward a further education.

Pain protection: You need to take care of your pain first. You would never be able to concentrate with all the pain you have. You would just embarrass yourself. First things first: Take care of your pain, and then you can go to school.

Who won the move? It sounds reasonable to take care of pain first. Pain wins.

Valued action: I want to meet someone and have an intimate relationship.

Pain protection: Who would want a person with chronic pain? You're not normal. Get rid of the pain first, and then maybe you would be acceptable.

Who won? Again, it sounds reasonable to first try to get rid of the pain in order to become more lovable and develop a relationship. Pain wins.

Valued action: I'm tired of being on disability. I want to get out and work and feel that I'm a part of society.

Pain protection: You can do that as soon as you get rid of this pain. What employer wants a person who suffers from chronic pain? You need to get healthy first, and then think about a job.

Who won? The fear of not being acceptable and possibly being rejected steers the move toward controlling and protecting the pain. Pain wins.

Final score: 3 to 0. Pain wins.

As you can see from this example, the pain team is winning all the major battles and gaining position and the values team is losing territory. Is this what's happening to you? This is the scenario for most people who live with chronic pain. Pain and trying to cope with pain occupy more and more realms of life until it feels they must be considered at all times in all situations.

EXERCISE: YOUR BATTLE BETWEEN LIVING A VALUED LIFE AND PROTECTING YOURSELF FROM PAIN

Think about one of the struggles you've had within yourself between the pain side and the valued life side of this battle. Describe what the struggle was about and which side won. Doing this exercise can help you to see how your mind sometimes fights against itself.

Valued action: _____

_____

_____

_____

_____

Pain protection: _____

_____

_____

_____

_____

_____

Result: _____

_____

_____

_____

_____

_____

Being the Pieces

Like most people, you probably get involved in these battles and try to help one side or the other win. One day you may decide you'll join the "good" side (living a valued life), so you jump on your horse ready to battle for your values despite your pain. On other days you probably join the side that's trying to protect you from pain. In the latter case, you genuinely believe that you need to heal your chronic pain before you can make the moves in life that you most want to make.

No doubt, you win some of these battles. Some days you move in the directions you value, and some days you successfully protect yourself from pain. But are you really going anywhere while stuck in this battle? Are you really making any moves that take you to a place you want to be in the long run?

And besides, where are *you* in this eternal battle anyway? Where are you in this ongoing battle between the life you want to live and the pain you're trying to avoid? Which part of this game is about you? This is an actual question. Where are *you* in all this? Write your answer in the space below.

Did you say that you're the white side fighting for your valued life? Did you say you're the black side, trying to stave off pain? But don't you contain both sides of the battle? What does it mean if you are either the white pieces or the black pieces? You can take sides, and you can win a battle here and there, but are you ever going to win this war? Probably not. Think about who is battling whom here. Every single one of the pieces on this chessboard belongs to you, and when you go to war against yourself, you always lose. Pain is a significant part of who you are. If you regard it as the enemy, every time you fight with it you're fighting yourself. Every time you beat it, you're beating yourself. In this battle you always lose, because every player in the battle is part of who you are. If pain is your enemy and fighting is your only option, you are permanently stuck living in a war zone, and that's no way to live your life.

But maybe you aren't the pieces. Maybe you aren't the white side or the black side. Could that be possible? And if it is, then what are you?

Being the Chessboard

ACT posits that you are the chessboard (Hayes, Strosahl, and Wilson 1999). You're not either the white side or the black side; you're the white side *and* the black side (and every side and angle in between for that matter). Becoming the observer self means looking at your life from the perspective of the chessboard, not from the perspective of the pieces.

Being the chessboard offers you a way to step out of the war with your pain that you've been in for so long. Instead of being the pieces, you contain the pieces. Instead of fighting in a battle, you are the ground on which the battle is fought. Looking at your life from this perspective is what we call "being mindful." Although it might be interpreted as such, being mindful doesn't mean being full of your mind. It doesn't mean looking at your life from your mind's eye. It means looking at your life from your observer self. It means learning to see that the pieces of you that are battling on and on are only part of what you are. You can learn to watch this battle without attachment to it. You can learn to be mindful.

In fact, the more you try to look at your life from this perspective, the easier mindfulness becomes. Practice doesn't make perfect—it makes permanent. What we mean by that is that you need to practice being mindful in order to be mindful. The rest of this chapter is dedicated to teaching you how to practice mindfulness. We'll guide you through some specific exercises you can employ to take this practice with you outside the confines of this book and into your real life.

THE PRACTICE OF MINDFULNESS

Despite the fact that there are techniques that help you become more mindful, mindfulness is not some special mystical state that you enter into. Mindfulness simply involves learning to operate more and more from the perspective of your observer self—the self that's with you every moment of your life. So being mindful isn't anything special; it's really the most fundamental way of being in the world. That being said, when you first start to practice mindfulness, there are some parameters you need to consider.

When to Practice

Ultimately, you'll want to practice mindfulness whenever you are, wherever you are, and at any given point in time. But when you're first starting, it's a good idea to set up a schedule for your mindfulness practice. If you promise yourself that you'll practice when you remember to, it's likely that you won't practice at all. We recommend that you commit to a specific schedule of mindfulness practice.

Start by practicing for at least half an hour two to three times a week. If this is absolutely not possible for you, try to work up to this level of practice. Over time, try to work up to daily practice if you can. This may sound like a lot of time, but think about how much time you spend struggling with your pain right now. If you were to estimate the amount of time you spend thinking about, battling, or trying to get rid of your pain, do you think it would come to more than three and a half hours per week? That's all the time we're asking you to dedicate to this practice, which just might help you live a better quality of life with your pain than you ever have before.

During your practice sessions, work with any or all of the techniques in this chapter. If you find other techniques that work for you, include those as well. There are no limitations on how you can practice mindfulness, so try as many approaches as you wish.

In addition to your scheduled practice, don't rule out the possibility of practicing at random times throughout the day when the opportunity presents itself (and the opportunity is always present). Mindfulness shouldn't be relegated to the half hour you've scheduled to spend on it, so practice throughout your day, too. You'll find that this becomes more and more natural over time.

Where to Practice

You need not lock yourself in a room and demand total silence in order to practice mindfulness. Being mindful isn't about eliminating distractions or obstacles, it's about seeing them for what they are. But when you're just starting to look at your thoughts as thoughts, it can sometimes be difficult to see, hear, or feel them if you're distracted by your children wrestling in the living room or if you're worried that your boss is going to walk in on your practice at work. In time you'll learn to take mindfulness with you everywhere you go, but for starters, figure out a good place to practice at the same time you decide when you'll practice.

How to Practice

The only thing you need to do when you practice being mindful is simply be in the observer self's seat and watch what comes up for you. Some of the things that come up will be good, some will be bad. Sometimes you'll have pain, sometimes you won't. Sometimes you'll think you really have this whole mindfulness thing nailed, and sometimes you'll feel so distracted you might wonder if you're losing your mind. (By the way, losing your mind isn't such a bad thing, so don't worry too much about it.)

When you practice mindfulness, you aren't trying to evoke some peaceful or beatific state. You're just looking at what happens for you from a perspective that you've been looking from throughout your life. The only difference is that now you're consciously engaging in the act of watching.

As mentioned above, sometimes you'll feel like you are really being mindful and sometimes you'll feel like you can't do this "mindfulness thing" at all. Remember, this is all just more content that your mind is producing for you. Mindfulness isn't a new measure for assessing success or failure. In fact, mindfulness isn't about success or failure at all. If you fall into the content your mind provides for you, if you start getting caught up in your pain, your thoughts about pain, or anything else for that matter (like whether you want eggs or pancakes for breakfast), just look at this as another opportunity to practice consciously observing your experience from the perspective of your observer self. Notice that you've fallen into your content, and then gently bring yourself back into the observer's seat.

By the way, you'll never get to a place where you are mindfully defused from your thoughts, feelings, and bodily sensations at all times. Doing that would be useless, anyway. You need to be able to slip into your conceptualized self from time to time. This is a natural facet of the human experience, and we aren't encouraging you to eliminate it. Rather, we want to help you broaden your resources by teaching you how to develop mindfulness. With that in mind, let's move on to the exercises.

EXERCISE: BEING IN THE MOMENT

In this exercise you're going to take a few moments to fully, consciously, mindfully be in the present moment (Hayes, Strosahl, and Wilson 1999). This exercise is essentially a dialogue. It's a set of verbal instructions built to help you become mindfully aware of your surroundings and your internal content. To do the exercise, simply follow the instructions below. If you wish, you can tape-record these instruction so you can play them back to yourself during your mindfulness training sessions. Other options are simply to read the instructions while you do the exercise or to memorize the basic components of the exercise and implement them on your own. Whatever method you choose, the practice is essentially the same. Let's get started.

Where are you in this moment? Take a moment to look around at your surroundings. What do you see? Is there anything that catches your eye? If so, just take note of it. Look at the desk, the plant, the bed, the stove, the tabletop, the tree, the sky, the waterfall, whatever is in your surroundings. Just look at it. See it and let it go. Watch yourself watching your surroundings.

What do you hear? Stretch out with your ears. Bring your attention to your hearing. What sounds do you hear? Is there anything you hear that draws you to it? What is it? Take note of it. Listen to it. Just be mindful of the sound. Is it a beautiful sound or an ugly sound? How does the sound make you feel? It doesn't have to make you feel any particular way, but if it does, note that too, then move on.

Think about smell. What can you smell in the place you're sitting or lying or standing in? Do you smell anything at all? Does that smell bring up any associations for you? What does it bring up? Note what it brings up without getting attached to it. If you feel yourself slip off into a memory or a fantasy, gently bring yourself back to the present moment. You are right here, right now practicing mindfulness.

Gradually bring your attention to your body. How does your body feel? Is it loose or tight? Are there particular areas of your body you're especially aware of? Rub your fingertips together. What is that like? Can you feel your fingerprints? Are your fingers rough or smooth? Do you need to moisturize? If you're sitting in something or lying on something, think about how that feels. Turn your attention to where your body meets whatever it is you're resting on. At the point of contact between your body and this surface, what do you experience? Simply note the experience. Is it pleasurable? Is the chair or the bed soft or rough? Do you feel pressure on parts of your body? Where is this pressure? What is it like? Try not to fall into what your body is experiencing. Just look at it and let it go.

Now try to bring your attention to your pain. Don't worry; you're just going to have a look at it. See if you can contact it without becoming attached to it. Where do you feel pain? Try to be specific if you can. How does it feel? Is it a long, dull ache or a sharp stab? Note how much your experience of pain can vary. See if it changes while you look at it. Does the pain move around in your body? See where it goes and just make note of it. If you fall into how badly you hurt from time to time, that's okay. Just bring yourself gently back to this moment and know that the you who is always you is just watching your pain. No problem there. You are just watching the pain. See it. Feel it. Hear it. Try not to attach to it. It is there. It is part of you, just like your toes or your fingers.

When you're done looking at your pain, see if you have any thoughts, feelings, or memories coming to your consciousness. If you do, note them. What do you feel now? Are you scared because of having come in contact with your pain? If so, just note that feeling. You might tell yourself, "This is me feeling that I'm scared." Are you feeling angry that this exercise is making you come in contact with your pain? You can just look at that, too. This is all more content that your mind is producing. Remember, you are the chessboard. Each of these feelings is just a piece of you.

Now turn to your thoughts. Are there any thoughts coming up for you in this moment? What are they? Listen to them as they are spoken in your mind. What are they saying? What kind of information is your mind rattling off today? Listen to it the way you might listen to a radio. There it is, going on and on. But the you that is you is there just listening.

You can handle any memories that come up when you do this exercise in the same way. There's no need to go out and look for them. Just let them rise and fall away like waves on the ocean. They come in, and then they dissipate. You breathe them in; you exhale them out. You are not attached to your memories. If you fall into one and find yourself in the memory instead of in the present moment, that isn't a problem. Just note what has happened and resume the observer's seat.

You can carry on with this exercise as long as you wish, noting whatever is around and within you. When you feel you are finished, simply go on about your day. This was a moment. There are more moments to be had. Move on with your life.

If you wish, you can take some notes on this experience in the space below. If you want to take notes each time you practice, consider getting a journal for this purpose.

_____

_____

_____

_____

_____

MINDFUL JOURNALING

In this exercise we ask that you journal mindfully. To do so, get into the observer's seat and then take some time to write out whatever comes up for you. You can write out every thought, every feeling, every bodily sensation. It doesn't matter what you write. It doesn't have to be connected to anything. There is no theme, and what you write need not have any continuity. This is simply you watching yourself produce verbal content in a form that is very close to being a direct transcription of what your mind is doing in the moment. This is your mind at work. This is you watching your mind at work.

You can write anything that comes into your head. You can write about the stove top or the cat. You can write about how you were ashamed to be scared when you walked outside in the middle of the night to bring the garbage cans around to the front of the house. You can write about your pain. You can write about how much it hurts. You can write about how much you battle with it. No matter what the topic, just write and write and write. After all, this is what your mind is doing anyway, isn't it? In this exercise you're just giving voice to your mind.

Try to remain mindful as you write. Sometimes you'll sink into the content on the page. That's okay. It happens. Just bring yourself back to the present moment. Watch the pen move in your hand. Watch how it scratches out inky symbols that are mere representations of what you think. Just sit and write and watch yourself writing. Allow it to happen naturally and without any interruption. And when you are done, stop.

_____

_____

_____

_____

_____

_____

_____

_____

_____

_____

_____

_____

_____

_____

_____

_____

_____

_____

_____

_____

_____

_____

Again, this is a practice you can institute as much and as often as you like. You can get a journal and keep your mindful journaling in it if you wish. Better yet, simply pick up a tablet of paper, journal mindfully, and then set it free when you're done. You can tear it up, throw it away, or burn it. This isn't done in the spirit of destruction. You aren't try to kill your thoughts or break your mind; rather, it's done in the spirit of learning to let go.

SITTING PRACTICE

The final form of mindfulness practice we'll introduce you to in this chapter is sitting practice. This is a form of mindfulness training developed in Eastern cultures and refined over thousands of years. In essence the practice is very simple. Just sit. That's all: you simply sit. However, in daily practice it's a little more complicated than this. This probably isn't the first time you've encountered that simple things can be the most difficult.

Sitting practice isn't meditation. It isn't some mystical form of heightened awareness or a special spiritual practice (at least it doesn't need to be). It's an opportunity to be still and watch what your mind produces for you.

There are a few things you need to consider so that you can develop a powerful sitting practice.

When and Where

As with the other mindfulness exercises in this chapter, you need to develop a consistent regimen of practice. Decide when you're going to sit and where you're going to sit, and then do it. There will always be reasons not to do sitting practice. Making a commitment to practice is the best way to develop your mindfulness skills.

The Posture

Many books have addressed the posture you should take while you sit. You can either sit on a pillow on the ground or sit in a chair. If you sit on the ground, there are various cross-legged positions you can assume based on how advanced you are in your practice. We won't elaborate on this here, but if you're interested you can refer to *The Relaxation and Stress Reduction Workbook* (Davis, Eshelman, and McKay 2000) for more information on the various postures you can assume when seated on the ground.

Wherever and however you sit, make sure your back is straight and relaxed. If you sit in a chair, don't lean back against the chair and slump. Sit on the front two-thirds of the chair and try not to rest your back against the chair at all. Maintain good posture. This means that the crown of your head should be reaching toward the sky and your lower back should be straight, or slightly arched so that it pushes your stomach forward a bit.

Rest your hands in your lap, or form them into a "mudra," wherein your fingers overlap and your thumbs touch slightly to make a circle.

Once you've assumed this posture, try not to break it for the duration of your practice session. To help with this, make sure you've assumed a stable, steady posture before the session actually begins.

How

When you sit, you need to be still and quiet for the amount of time you've specified for your practice. This means you should move as little as possible while you sit. Over time, you may feel that the position you're sitting in is uncomfortable. This is almost universally true for people who do a sitting practice. You won't be comfortable all the time; that simply isn't human nature. Accept your discomfort as part of the practice. Don't squirm around or change positions unless you absolutely have to. When that happens, simply shift your position and go back to sitting. If you come to a point where you feel discomfort, look at it as a way to deepen your practice. The truth is, it's often easier to practice being mindful when conditions aren't challenging. To really develop your mindfulness skills, you need to practice through the difficult times. Take advantage of them.

In fact, precisely because you struggle with chronic pain, taking the time to try to sit with your pain will be a very valuable practice for you. If you stop sitting or get up and move around each time you feel uncomfortable, you're setting a dangerous precedent for yourself that very well may spill over into your daily life. When you practice sitting with pain and discomfort, you afford yourself the opportunity to expand the way you handle pain in your daily life. Do your best.

That being said, this is not a time to grit your teeth and bear it. Be gentle and compassionate with yourself as well. Although you should try hard to sit with the pain, if you can't endure it, give yourself a break and try again next time. Your struggle with pain is an ongoing, ever-changing process, as is life itself. If you don't "get it" this time, you'll have other opportunities to do so. Practice is just that: practice.

Other than that, all you need to do is mindfully watch what comes up for you while you sit. Use the skills you've learned thus far in the book, become the chessboard, and simply watch what the pieces do. Sometimes you will fall into the battle. Sometimes you'll become one of the pieces. Sometimes your pain will take over. Again, that's okay. When these things happen, just bring yourself back to the present moment and go back to your sitting practice until the session is finished.

And that's it: just sit. Watch your thoughts, feelings, and bodily sensations come in and go out with your breath. Feel your body, the room around you, and the world this room is in. Allow yourself to stretch out in your mind and let go. Sink into your humanness. Being mindful is your birthright as a human being. Take advantage of it.

MINDFULNESS AND ACCEPTANCE

Mindfulness is a powerful technique. It has the ability to change your perspective on the very nature of your humanity and on the pain you've been suffering from. But that's only part of the picture. Changes in perspective are good, but this book is about living your life. We want you to be able to take what's in this book and go out into the world vitalized and engaged in a life that reflects your true values.

In order to get to that place, there are some more steps to take. In the next chapter, you'll apply your new mindfulness skills to find ways you can accept your pain so you can live with it instead of in opposition to it. This is where we start to pick up speed. You have the basic techniques down; now it's time to advance into the final steps of this program. Acceptance is at its very core. So if you're ready to take a leap into a new life, dive into the next chapter to learn more about how you can develop acceptance.

CHAPTER 6

Are You Willing?

Part of the reason that moving into the position of the observer self is so powerful is because you start to see that the you that is always you is not bound by any single element of your private experience. You may think or feel many different things, but those feelings and ideas don't define who you are. You contain them, but you aren't limited by them. It allows you to see that your struggle with chronic pain need not define you. It is a part of your experience, but it isn't your only experience. You have pain, but you are not the pain. This gives you more maneuvering room in life than you had before. This doesn't mean the pain goes away. Becoming mindful doesn't get rid of pain, and it isn't a way to escape from your personal experience, but it does allow you to see your pain in the larger context of your total being. The pain itself remains; it is your perspective on it that changes.

Has this shift begun to occur for you? In the previous two chapters we worked on taking distance from your thoughts and feelings about pain and getting into the role of the observer self. By now you may have started to open up to a new sense of who you are as a person. You may now be able to look *at* your thoughts, feelings, and bodily sensations rather than *from* them. You may start to see your experience with pain in a different light.

When you come into contact with your observer self, the continuous thread of your being, your perspective on how much pain dominates your existence changes.

If you've started to get a sense of this, then you're ready to take the next step in your journey toward living the valued life you've been dreaming of. It is one of the most important steps you'll take in this book, and it is also one of the most healing. That step is acceptance.

ACCEPTANCE: A BOLD STEP TOWARD A VALUED LIFE

Can you imagine a life where pain is not an obstacle to moving in the direction you want to move in? What if you could start living your life the way you want to live it right now, with your pain along for the ride? In chapter 3 you explored your values and how you most want to be living right now; you developed a greater understanding of the life that would fill you up and give you vitality. Rather than waiting for your pain to go away so that you can start living that life, what if there were a move you could make that would allow you to start down that path right now, today, this very moment? Indeed, there is, and that move is called acceptance.

For the purposes of this book, we define acceptance as the act by which you allow yourself to willingly engage your pain. Unfortunately, in our culture, when people hear a statement like that they often think it means all sorts of things it doesn't mean. After reading that statement, you may be cringing in your chair. You may be thinking, "Great, after all this they're going to tell me to give up and just accept my pain." But what we suggest you try is totally different than giving up. Acceptance is an active, positive, engaged embracing of your experience undertaken so that you can more fully live your life (Hayes, Strosahl, and Wilson 1999). Let us explain.

Giving up and just accepting that you can't do anything about your pain or your life is what we would call "passive resignation." This state of mind is not a reflection of giving up the struggle with pain, it's a reflection of giving in to the struggle. In this defeatist stance, you just let the pain win because you think there's nothing else you can do. When you "accept" in this fashion, you're still caught on the level of the chess pieces. You're still mired in the struggle between having pain and living a life that you value. Even if you give up and let the black side win, you've still engaged in the game. This is not what acceptance is about.

Acceptance is about getting into the perspective of the observer self—being the chessboard, not the pieces—and making an active choice to accept that which cannot be changed. You probably know by now that you aren't going to be able to win your battle with pain. Even if we haven't successfully convinced you of that in this book, your own experience has probably been hinting at that conclusion for some time. You've tried the therapies. You've tried the medications. You've tried suppressing the pain. You may feel as though you've tried everything. And there it is, your pain, still ominous, haunting, and ever present. So if you can't get rid of it, what would accepting it do for you? What would it be like if you were finally to come to terms with the fact that the pain isn't going away? What if you were to open your arms and embrace the pain warmly, as a part of who you are as a human being? Would it change the way pain operated for you?

Acceptance has gotten a bad reputation in this culture, so we often refer to acceptance as "willingness" in the ACT community. You will find these two terms used interchangeably throughout the rest of this book.

Despite its relatively poor reputation, the merits of acceptance are revealed in various idiomatic phrases and wise sayings in our culture. You often hear people saying things like, "She simply can't accept [whatever], and that's why she continues to have these problems." The problem is that we generally don't take these turns of phrase all that seriously anymore. That's unfortunate, because if we heard them or saw them for what they really mean, they have the power to unveil some of the truth about acceptance. An excellent example is the serenity creed we introduced you to back in chapter 2. Here it is again, as a refresher: Grant me the courage to change the things I can, the serenity to accept the things I cannot change, and the wisdom to know the difference.

You undoubtedly had heard the serenity creed before you ever opened this book. Upon encountering the phrase "Grant me the serenity to accept the things I cannot change," you may even have thought, "If only I could do that." But then you probably let it go and reengaged in your daily battle with pain unaware that you *can* develop acceptance in regard to your pain. You can learn to be willing to have your pain. It's in your power to develop the skills to do so. We'll help you learn some of those techniques in this chapter, but there are a few more issues we need to address first.

Why Accept?

At this point, you're probably wondering why we suggest you accept your pain. And that is an excellent question. One simple answer may be, "Why not?" After all, you've tried just about everything else. You might as well give acceptance a shot and see if it works out for you. If it does, great; you'll have a new way to understand your current dilemma. If it doesn't, at least you gave it a shot.

Beyond this, there are other reasons you might want to learn to accept your pain. ACT is ultimately a pragmatic therapeutic approach. That means we encourage people to make choices based on practical outcomes. The way that ACT therapy is constructed reflects this to some degree. With ACT, the issue isn't whether or not you can come to some profound or mystical insight about the nature of your pain and your experience in life. At its root, it's about how you live your life day to day.

This is why we spend so much time asking people to investigate their values. Your values are a practical tool you can use to build your life into what you want it to be, and we'll teach you more about that in the next chapter. But on that road to your valued life, there are inevitably obstacles. There you are, walking down your valued path, and *boom!* Out of nowhere, here comes your chronic pain. It's a big beast that blocks your path, and it's scary. It has sharp teeth that cut into your tender spots every time you encounter it. You were having a nice hike down this beautiful path toward the life you always wanted to live, and then, out of nowhere, you find yourself in pain. Now what? If you have to stop and wrestle this beast to the ground every time you face it on your path, you aren't going to make much forward progress.

But what if you were to invite the beast to come along with you? What if you were to turn to this beast and ask it to come along with you, with all its horrible beastliness, with its sharp, biting teeth. You've run across this beast so many times, why not just invite it along for the ride this time?

In ACT, we use a metaphor about a guy some people would call beastly. His name is Joe the Bum, and we'd like to tell you about him now (Hayes, Strosahl, and Wilson 1999).

Joe the Bum

Imagine that you've planned an open house cocktail party in your home. You've sent out invitations to everyone in the neighborhood and put up some flyers. You've been planning this party for months so every detail will be perfect. You've got the perfect china, you've made the perfect food, and you've bought the perfect wine. You really want this night to be special. You've wanted to offer this kind of hospitality to the people in your neighborhood for a long time, so you intend to make an evening of it.

You have an image in your head of the perfect party, with well-behaved guests. They all dress in a certain way, and they all act according to the social conventions of a cocktail party. All the guests show up as planned, and they mingle exactly as you had pictured. It looks as though it's going to turn out to be a beautiful night.

Then, all of a sudden, you hear a loud banging on the door. You shudder to think who it might be. Even though you said everyone was invited to your party, the fact is, you didn't mean *everyone*. You really only wanted those people whom you knew would fit into your picture of the perfect party. You certainly didn't want Joe the Bum to show up. This guy is a menace. He smells bad, he wears ratty clothes, and the worst part is that he harasses everyone in the neighborhood. He walks up and down the streets, and whenever he sees someone, he starts giving them mean looks and talking badly about them. You really don't like Joe the Bum. You even had the cops come pick him up one night to take him away, but he came back. This guy doesn't seem to be leaving your neighborhood anytime soon, and what's worse, here he is at your door on this special evening.

So whether you like it or not, Joe the Bum is on your doorstep. Next thing you know, he's in your house. Tonight he's way over the top. He must have been drinking before he showed up. He's annoyingly boisterous, he's making lewd and obnoxious comments to your guests, and his ragged clothes smell worse than usual. You're completely shocked and overwhelmed by his presence. This is not how you wanted this night to turn out.

At first you spend every moment trying to figure out ways to contain him in certain areas, trying to hide him. Eventually you can't take it anymore, and you start arguing with him openly, telling him to leave. You yell at him that he had no right to show up at your doorstep and tell him how much you hate him. Joe doesn't seem to care all that much. He's just there for the party. You try giving up and letting him stay, but you just can't manage to do it.

Over the course of the evening, you lose sight of your party and your guests altogether as you focus on controlling Joe. But Joe is impossible to control and your party turns into a disaster, so you ask everyone to go home. They do, and you're left sitting with Joe in the kitchen at the end of the evening. You start crying and accusing Joe of ruining your cocktail party with his inappropriate behavior. Joe just turns to you and says, "But you said everyone was welcome." You respond by saying, "Yes, I did say that, but I expected people to come who know how to behave properly in a social situation."

Then Joe lets the bomb fall. He tells you that he's always going to show up, especially when and where you least want him to. He says that he doesn't have any intention of leaving or letting things be easy for you, so you might as well give that up right now.

As Joe is talking, you begin to realize that the whole night you were focused on controlling Joe. And as long as you did that, you couldn't pay attention to your guests and enjoy the party. In fact, the party disappeared for you the moment you started spending all your energy on trying to get Joe under control.

You and Joe talk about this problem you're having with one another and come up with a few possible solutions together:

1. Teach Joe to behave properly first, then have parties.

2. Numb yourself from reacting to Joe by using drugs or alcohol.

3. Avoid Joe altogether by not having or attending any more parties.

4. Suppress your reactions to Joe by keeping yourself busy.

5. Accept Joe completely, just as he is—with his smelly clothes and his bad attitude—*and* enjoy your party.

Which of these alternatives would you choose? _____

The first four options ultimately mean that you aren't going to be able to enjoy yourself when Joe's around. The first option looks tempting. You want to get Joe under control before you have any more parties. But deep down you know that Joe is a hopeless case. He himself has said that he doesn't want to change and doesn't want to make it easy on you. Given that, how could you possibly train him to be socially appropriate? Even if you did take the time and had some success in training him, wouldn't you then have to keep an eye on him throughout any future parties? That doesn't sound like much fun.

If you try to numb yourself to Joe's presence with drugs or alcohol, you know what the effects will be. You may be able to ignore him for a while, but in your numbed state, you're going to miss most of the party, too, and in the end you're just going to have a headache and an upset stomach in the morning.

Not having or attending parties isn't much of an option. That just means you don't get to have any fun at all.

You could try to suppress your reactions to Joe by keeping yourself busy, but is that really all that different from drinking yourself numb? Either way, you miss the party.

The only way to enjoy your party is to accept Joe. There just isn't another way. It might be nice if there were, but that isn't the reality. Resisting, struggling with, or trying to control Joe doesn't get rid of him, and it takes you away from your fun. By accepting Joe's presence, you accept that you cannot control the inevitable imperfections, deviations, and unwanted feelings and thoughts. And at the same time, you get to enjoy the party you created. You can take the bad with the good and enjoy the time you have at the party.

This is the essence of acceptance: living with what you cannot control, even if it's unpleasant, *and* actively pursuing the life you want. Accepting Joe is the only way that you can have fun at your party. There are other things in your life like that, too. Now let's see what we can do about that other bum—your pain.

Why Accept—Revisited

The story of Joe the Bum probably gave you some hints about why accepting your pain may be something you want to engage in. The reason to accept—the big reason—is so that you can live the vital, engaged, meaningful life that you want to live starting right now, in this very moment. If you just accept that you can't get rid of Joe, *and* at the same time you continue with the party just as you would have, then you can have fun.

The same is true of your life. How many times have you stopped on your valued path to wrestle your pain monster to the ground? How far do you get before the monster is right there in your path again? How many times has Joe interfered in your life?

Take a moment to look back at your values compass in chapter 3. If you aren't clear about how many times pain has been an obstacle on your path to a valued life, examine the discrepancies between where you are right now on your valued path and where you want to be. What's been holding you back?

Everything in your experience up to this point has been telling you that there are aspects of your life that you can't change and that your pain is one of them. You can compare yourself to other people, you can call it unfair, you can fight the pain, you can get involved with any of these pieces on the chessboard, but in the end none of that matters a great deal. You haven't been able to get rid of your pain, and it looks as though you might not be able to. So what are you going to do with it as long as you're stuck with it?

It's as though you have a radio that only has two dials on it (Hayes, Strosahl, and Wilson 1999). One dial reflects the amount of pain you'll feel throughout life. The second dial represents your ability to accept your pain. The dial for the amount of pain you experience lives its own life; you have no control over it. You know this, because you've been trying to control it for a long time. You turn it down and it springs back up. You ignore it, but it turns itself up to get your attention. Sometimes it just goes up and down for no apparent reason whatsoever. You can't really influence what it does.

On the other hand, the dial that reflects your willingness to accept your pain is a dial you have complete control over. How willing you are to accept your pain is entirely your choice. You can set the dial high and choose a life that is full of acceptance, or you can set the dial low and choose a life of struggle. That choice is yours.

You may have begun to experience this somewhat indirectly as you worked through the previous two chapters. When you choose to willingly sit with your pain, you make a choice to turn your acceptance dial up and ignore the pain dial (Hayes, Strosahl, and Wilson 1999).

There's something else you may have noticed. When you turn down the acceptance dial and say something like "I can't stand the pain," you spring-load the pain dial and it shoots sky-high. That is to say, when you refuse to accept, you end up in even more pain than when you choose to accept. This ultimately goes back to the discussion of experiential avoidance earlier in the book. Each and every time you tell yourself that you can't accept your pain, you're actually calling your pain to mind. And each time you call your pain to your conscious mind, it simply reinforces the pain itself, as well as the power the pain has over your life.

There is a saying in ACT that reflects this phenomenon quite nicely: If you don't want it, you've got it (Hayes, Strosahl, and Wilson 1999). Every time you turn down your acceptance dial, you end up with the very pain that you were trying to escape in the first place.

When you turn up the acceptance dial, something entirely different happens. Your pain may stay or it may leave, but you don't get caught up trying to control things that you can't control. Instead, you use your time and energy to build the life you want to live. That means that you can still keep moving in your valued directions no matter what happens with the pain dial. When you turn up your acceptance dial and invite your pain monster to come along with you, you can move forward with or without it; its presence matters little.

This may sound pretty good to you right now. In fact, it might sound too good to be true. Don't worry, acceptance can work for you, but it's good for you to bring your skeptical mind along with you for the ride as there are some pitfalls to acceptance. However, these pitfalls might not be exactly where you think they are. So before you continue down this path of acceptance, let's have a look at the pitfalls so you can be aware of them in advance.

Acceptance Pitfalls

Right now you are probably thinking that acceptance sounds like it just might be a good idea. You think that if you practice acceptance, then you'll be able to live the life you want to live. That sounds fairly rational, so you think you'll try acceptance. Don't be confused. This is *not* how acceptance works.

Reconsider the concept that if you practice acceptance, then you'll be able to live the life you want to live. Doesn't it sound like some of the other statements and rationalizations that your mind tries to give you? Here are a few examples: "If I get rid of my pain, then I can live my life." "If I stop feeling so bad, then I'll do what I want to do." "If I can get rid of Joe, then I'll have a party." With these types of statements, your mind is trying to trick you into operating on its level. However, operating on that level completely disempowers your acceptance work. This goes back to a recurring theme we've addressed in this book: experiential avoidance.

In the mindfulness exercises you've been practicing, you may have noticed that when you are fully in the observer's seat—when you become the chessboard and just watch the players play—your direct experience with pain diminishes. It seems as though the pain goes down for a while. This nice little side effect of mindfulness and acceptance techniques is fine in a way, but it's also a little dangerous. The reason it's dangerous is because your mind starts to see this process at work and tells you that acceptance is a good idea, since it makes the pain go away. When the pain goes away, you can live the life you want, so acceptance makes rational sense and you should try it. This message from your mind is one of the same old traps that your mind has been laying for you all along, and buying into it puts you right back in the world of experiential avoidance.

Once you start accepting to keep your pain at bay, then you aren't really accepting at all. You are just using acceptance as a way of avoiding your experience with pain. This is not what we mean by acceptance. Acceptance has to be done fully, with an open mind and an open heart. If you're trying to accept for "reasons," then you aren't accepting at all. Acceptance allows you the space to live the life you want to live, but only if you open up your arms as wide as they can go for a full-body embrace of your pain.

This leads us to the second major pitfall that you may find on the road to acceptance: You can't try to accept. You either choose to accept or you don't. Upon hearing about acceptance, many people say, "Well, I guess I'll give it a try." But acceptance simply does not function this way. You must entirely commit to the process of acceptance; there's no middle path. Although you can limit when you're willing to feel pain and how long you're willing to feel pain in a given situation (distinctions that we will explore more later in the chapter), you can't limit your level of acceptance.

The concept that you can't *try* to accept may seem a little confusing, but there are actually many other aspects of human existence that are very much like this. For example, reach out and try to touch your skin. Don't actually touch it; just *try* to touch it. Can you do this? No, you can't. You can either touch your skin or not touch your skin, but there's no way to *try* to touch your skin. It's simply a choice that you make, and then you implement that choice.

Another example is jumping: You could jump off a chair, out of your window, off your roof, out of a plane. You have some choice about where you jump from, but if you make the choice to jump there's no trying involved. You just jump. Acceptance must be approached in this same spirit (Hayes, Strosahl, and Wilson 1999). Give up trying and just do it. There's no other way to accept.

Now that you're aware of the potential pitfalls, it's time for you to make a choice. Are you willing to accept your pain, or aren't you?

Making the Vital Embrace: Accepting Your Pain

It's one thing to encounter acceptance incidentally through defusion and mindfulness exercises. Those exercises are important aspects of this program, and they'll serve you well on your road to acceptance. But to truly accept, you need to make a conscious decision that you will accept your pain. Now is the time to make that decision.

We pose this question to you: Are you ready to take a big step and willingly embrace your pain, looking at it from the perspective of your observer self, seeing it as it is and not as it says it is, in order to live the valued life you've always wanted to live?

Yes or No?

If you answered no, look at why you answered that way and ask yourself what your answer is in the service of. Is there any way that you might be able to change your answer? What would doing that cost you? What might it allow you to achieve? If you still can't come to a resounding yes, you might consider reviewing the earlier chapters in this book. Working on your mindfulness and defusion skills may help you see a way that you can open up and embrace your pain.

If you answered yes from your whole being, not just with your brain, and you're ready to embrace that part of you that is your pain, good for you! You've taken an important step on your journey to your valued life, and you're ready to learn how to apply this full embrace in your everyday life. The rest of this chapter is designed to help you do just that.

ACCEPTANCE EVERY DAY

Each new day offers you the opportunity to engage in acceptance and to accept your pain. It isn't always easy; in fact, it won't be easy most of the time. But with time and practice you can learn how to openly embrace your pain even in the most difficult situations.

The first step is to get into the observer's seat when you encounter situations that require acceptance. When you operate from your observer self, you can see your life more completely and you can more clearly determine how acceptance serves your whole self. When you're in your conceptualized self—when you get caught up on the level of the chess pieces—it's much more difficult to open up and accept your experience as it is and not as what it says it is.

This is why we guided you through exercises on defusion and mindfulness before tackling acceptance. The strategies you learned in those exercises are the foundation for your acceptance work. Don't forget them, and always take them with you. They are your tools now, and you can use them as you choose. Place yourself in the observer's seat and explore the following exercises, all of which will help you practice acceptance.

EXERCISE: TURNING UP THE ACCEPTANCE DIAL

Remember the metaphor of the radio with two dials that we referred to earlier? In this exercise, we'll teach you how to take this metaphor with you into your everyday life (Hayes, Strosahl, and Wilson 1999).

When you encounter what you perceive to be negative experiences, look at where your acceptance dial is set. As you'll recall, you have no control over your pain dial, so you might as well just leave that one where it is. But you have an amazing amount of control over your acceptance dial. Focusing on where that one is set can take you a long way toward your valued life.

When you come in contact with your pain and feel it's obstructing your life, look at your acceptance dial. If you notice it's set low, see if you can turn it up. Imagine there are tiny numbers on the dial, from 0 through 10; 0 indicates that you're totally unwilling to accept your pain, and 10 indicates that you're completely willing to accept your pain, whatever the circumstances. See if you can set your acceptance dial at 10 every time you come in contact with negative content. If you can't, ask yourself what setting the dial lower is in the service of. Take a step back, look at your thoughts, and see what they're telling you. Are you getting caught up in the games of your mind machine? If so, it's time to defuse and then see if you can set your acceptance dial at 10.

When you make this choice, keep a couple of things in mind. First, you can't try to accept. And second, you can't place a limit on the extent to which you're willing to accept. However, you can limit some of the practical parameters around your choice to be willing. For example, let's say that your child is having a dance recital and you really want to go, but you know it will last two hours and that sitting in a chair for that long will hurt your back. You want to go, yet you don't know if you can face the pain.

Take a step back and look at your thoughts and feelings about the event. Get into the observer's seat and take a moment to see what might be served by making the choice to accept your pain and go to the recital. If that choice supports your values and going to the recital is something that would make you feel vital and alive, then you know the choice comes down to either living a valued life or allowing your pain monster to obstruct that path once again.

In this situation, you might make this decision: "I'm going to turn my acceptance dial up to 10 for the duration of the recital. I'm going to embrace my pain and bring it along with me to my child's dance performance because being there is something that I value. But when the performance is over, I can choose to turn the dial back down, go home, and lie down for half an hour to give myself a break."

This is a perfectly valid way to use acceptance. When you choose to accept, you can accept for a limited time or in limited situations. With time and practice, you'll be able to build up to more and more acceptance. When you start, you may want to take bold steps, but don't make them so bold that they turn you off the idea of acceptance altogether.

So turn the dial up, but limit the amount of time or the situation in which you are going to leave it at a 10 if you need to. Then wake up the next day and see if you can turn it back up again.

EXERCISE: GIVING SHAPE TO YOUR PAIN— CREATING YOUR OWN PAIN MONSTER

Another thing you might do when you encounter pain in your daily life is to externalize it, give shape to it, and see if you can accept the pain monster you have created.

To do this, first try to come into conscious contact with your pain. Get into a mindful stance and see if you can contact your pain and look at it for what it is. Once you've done this, imagine how your pain might manifest if it were outside your body.

If you could put your pain outside your body, what shape would it have? _____

_____

_____

_____

If you could put your pain outside your body, how big would it be? _____

_____

_____

_____

What color would your pain be if it were outside your body? _____

_____

What texture would your pain have? Would it be rough or smooth, silky or like granite?

_____

_____

_____

If your pain had a voice, what would it sound like? _____

_____

_____

_____

How would your pain smell if it were outside your body? _____

_____

_____

_____

Now that you have your pain monster outside your body, take a look at it. What does it bring up for you? If it brings up negative thoughts, feelings, or bodily sensations, take those things and do the same exercise with them. If you have the feeling that you hate this pain monster, take that feeling, get it outside your body, and give it a shape, size, color, texture, voice, and smell. Now you have two monsters out there in front of you, or maybe more.

Now see if you can reach out and touch these monsters. See if you can gently stroke them on the surface of their bodies. Feel them as they are, not as they say they are.

When you're ready, see if you can accept these monsters exactly as you have created them. Try to take them back inside your body and gently store them where they were before. Remember, that place is your pain monster's home. If you don't allow it to be there, it may not have anywhere else to go. See if you can harbor these pain monsters the way you might harbor a lost and hurt child. Be gentle with them. Accept them. Hold them. They are your children after all.

GETTING BIGGER THAN YOUR PAIN

In the final acceptance exercise in this chapter, we want you to go out and actively seek your pain from the perspective of your observer self. This proactive way of accepting allows you the opportunity to chase down your pain and accept it, rather than waiting for it to ambush you.

To start, be seated, close your eyes, and take a deep breath. Take time to center yourself and notice your breathing. Passively let yourself be "breathed" and just let go. Relax and come into the observer's perspective.

Once you've done that, see if you can feel any tension or pain in your body. Are any of your regular aches and pains present in this moment? If they are, concentrate on that tension or pain and feel the energy it creates. Try to feel it as just energy. Be mindful and don't fall into one of your conceptualized selves.

Once you've come into contact with your pain and can feel the energy it's creating in your body, see if you can make room for that feeling of tension or pain. Let it be just where it is in this moment. If you want, you can put your hand on the part of your body where you feel the tension or pain. Just warm that place with your hand to mark where it is for yourself. See if you can open to your pain and accept it as just the feeling of energy that it's creating in that place in your body. You don't need to become attached to the pain. You can just accept it as it is and observe it.

Take some time to show your body compassion by noticing any bodily sensations you feel. Go through the different parts of your body, one by one, and check for any pain or tension. If you encounter pain or tension, go through the same process you did above: Feel it as energy and welcome it to stay just where it is. Tell your body that you accept and will make room for any feelings or sensations that are there, good or bad.

Start with your head, facial muscles, jaws, and neck. Let yourself feel each of these parts, and as you do so, think of how valuable each of these parts of your body is to you. Then move to your shoulders and note whether there's any tension or pain there. If there is, just allow yourself to go into that energy, feel what you feel, and accept it. Make room for each and every sensation without exception. If thoughts come into your head, just notice them as well and accept them as they are without buying into what they say.

If you fall into your mental content, come back to the present and focus on your body. Remember, it's your observer self who is making room for your pain and that you are much bigger than your pain. Now focus on your back. Feel the difference in the parts of your back that have contact with the chair and those parts that aren't in contact with it. Think of how valuable your back is to you. Think of all the work you've done in your life and all the fun you've had thanks to your strong back. Now make room for any unpleasant sensations in your back. This is part of the power your back has. Realize that your back needs care and attention to be able to continue to serve you the way you need it to. Give your back this attention right now. If you have any tension or pain in your back muscles, allow yourself to feel this sensation and then accept it. You can put your hand on any painful spots and send them warmth and attention.

Continue to your arms: elbows, forearms, wrists, and hands. Allow yourself to feel any tension and pain. Feel it fully and without resistance. Continue to your hips, thighs, knees, calves, ankles, and feet. As you observe each part of your body, check its status compassionately and allow yourself to feel any tension or pain. As you feel these problem places, just acknowledge them, let yourself feel the pain, and accept it.

When you've worked through your entire body in this way, slowly come back to the room you are sitting in right now, bringing with you all the achy energy in your body. To complete the exercise, take a walk around the room or around your neighborhood carrying your pain with you. Think of this as a symbol of how you intend to live your life—taking all aspects of your experience with you on the path of your valued life.

APPROACH PAIN AND DIFFICULT SITUATIONS WITH ACCEPTANCE

Now that you've learned some techniques to help you accept your pain and other adverse mental content when it comes up, we suggest that you actively and consciously put these exercises to work for you.

In the week to come, practice approaching your pain and other difficult situations with the acceptance techniques we've set forth in this chapter. Beyond that, try to actively and consciously engage in situations that may bring up pain for you. We're not asking you to seek out pain, per se, but rather to willingly engage in activities that are meaningful to you and that have brought on pain in the past. When you do, see if you can operate from the perspective of your observer self and accept your pain for what it is.

The aim of all of the exercises in this chapter is to help you to make the transition from struggling with your pain and difficult situations to approaching them with acceptance. Give this approach a fair chance so you can evaluate whether it helps you to come closer to the life you want to live.

To help you go out and test your acceptance skills against challenging situations you might actually encounter in your life, make a list of such situations in the space below. If you need a little help to get you going, take a look at the painful situations Beth came up with; her list appears after the blank form.

Your Stressful or Difficult Situations

Now, in the space below, make your own list of situations that are painful, stressful, or just difficult for you. As you do so, try to list situations that you're likely to experience this week. Then you can go out and look for them, and when you find them you can practice your new mindfulness and acceptance skills. In addition to listing situations that bring on physical pain, also include situations that might be psychologically distressing even if they're only indirectly related to your pain.

Situations that I expect will be physically painful:

- _____

- _____

- _____

- _____

- _____

- _____

- _____

Situations that are psychologically distressing:

- _____

- _____

- _____

- _____

- _____

- _____

Beth's Stressful or Difficult Situations

Here's Beth's list of difficult situations.

Situations that I expect will be physically painful:

- *Heavy household or gardening chores*

- *Going out to meet old friends*

- *Going out to exercise classes, and exercise in general*

- *Sitting through any of the kids' sports practices*

- *Helping my mother-in-law clean her apartment*

- *Washing the very dirty windows of our house*

- *Hosting our annual family get-together*

- *Playing with children on the playground*

- *Sitting through the lecture I've been wanting to attend*

Situations that are psychologically distressing:

- *The thought of going back to work*

- *Meeting with the insurance company to discuss my disability status*

- *Visiting work*

- *Talking to my neighbors about why I'm home from work*

- *Explaining to the kids why I can't do things with them like I used to*

- *Feeling guilty about not helping my mother-in-law, who just had a stroke*

- *Avoiding my husband when he wants to have sex*

- *Trying to explain to people what my problem is*

Once you've made your list, go out and try to consciously engage in these situations with acceptance and mindfulness. Keep in mind that you don't necessarily have to try the hardest one first (though you certainly could if you feel like you're ready for it). Rather, you can slowly build up your acceptance techniques by starting with easier situations and building up to increasingly difficult situations.

Now look back over your list and rate each item on a scale of 1 to 10, where 1 is hardly challenging at all and 10 is extremely challenging. Write your rating next to each situation on your list. Once you've quantified how challenging these situations are for you, you can construct a hierarchy that allows you to progress through the situations from least to most challenging.

Don't let this be an excuse to progress more slowly than need be. Although it can be good to start out with small steps, when you're ready (and you will know when you're ready), make the leap and see if you can engage in a painful situation that you rank as a 10 with mindfulness and acceptance.

Once you've gone out and engaged in some of your painful situations, you may want to take some notes on your experience. Use the space below to record your experience so you can continue to reflect on it and learn new ways to refine your acceptance techniques over time. You'll want to complete this analysis for all the situations you listed above, so make photocopies of this form rather than filling out the one in the book.

Difficult situation I engaged in:

_____

_____

_____

_____

What my mind and body were yelling at me (take notes on both your physical pain and what your mind wanted you to do about it):

_____

_____

_____

_____

My acceptance approach (what techniques you used and how they worked):

_____

_____

_____

_____

How I might refine my technique in the future (list any ways you think you might be more successful in practicing acceptance):

_____

_____

_____

_____

MOVING ON TO A VALUED LIFE

If you have learned to apply the techniques in this chapter, have made the conscious decision to accept, and have gone out and practiced your acceptance techniques in a variety of physically and psychologically painful situations, then your tool kit for living a valued life is almost complete. You have done some powerful work up to this point in the book, and you should be commended. Congratulations!

Now it is time to take the final step toward living your life the way you want to, bringing your pain along for the ride. In the next chapter you are going to generate a plan of committed action to put your valued life into play right now. You will be bringing everything you have learned in the book up to this point on the road with you, so don't forget these techniques. They are a powerful aid on this new road you are about to set out on.

CHAPTER 7

Committed Action

Imagine for a moment that you're a bus driver and that the destination sign on the front of your bus says "My Life" (Hayes, Strosahl, and Wilson 1999). You drive your route every day, and you stop at each stop along the way to collect passengers. Some of the passengers are friendly. Little old ladies sit at the front of your bus and chat with you as you drive along. Sometimes families climb aboard, the parents quiet with exhaustion, and the children rowdy with anticipation. You love each of these passengers and think of them as friends. You may not talk with all of them, but you see them every day and take them to their various destinations. You respect them and enjoy their presence.

But every once in a while, unpleasant and even heinous passengers climb on board your bus. Some of them are big and hairy and terrifying. Some are creepy creatures that wear black cloaks and have no faces. Your pain monster, which you met in the last chapter, gets on your bus every day. It doesn't always get on at the same stop, but somewhere along the line it gets on with its sharp, biting teeth that cause you so much distress.

Over time, it starts to feel as though the monsters are dominating the good passengers on your bus. They start moving to the front, and they tell your good passengers to squeeze into the back. Although your pain monster used to ride at the back of the bus, these days it sits right in the front, taking up as many seats as it pleases and telling the other passengers to go to hell if they don't like it. What's worse, these days it's barking orders at you and trying to tell you where to go. Because you're afraid of what this monster might do if you don't obey it, over the years you've started to listen to what it says and do what it wants.

As more time passes, you begin to realize that your bus doesn't follow its original route anymore. When you started driving the bus, you went in the direction you wanted to go. The passengers that came on just happened to be on that route. These days, you go where your pain monster tells you to go. It's bad enough that you don't get to drive where you want to anymore, but worse is that the beastly passengers are getting on your bus in ever-greater numbers these days, and they seem to be more awful than ever before. Nowadays you drive through parts of town where kind old ladies and families wouldn't dare to tread. Instead of your old, beloved passengers, monsters with ugly names like regret, loss, unhappiness, hopelessness, guilt, sorrow, and shame crowd onto your bus every day to ride with you.

Now, just for the sake of argument, let's say that one day you wake up and realize that you're actually still the driver of the bus and that it's still your choice where to go. The pain monster that has been with you so long had grown so loud (or maybe so quiet) that you became afraid of it, but that doesn't mean you can't change directions. You still control the direction and destination of your bus. You can take your bus wherever you want to go. The choice is yours.

So, armed with your new realization you get on the bus, and the first thing your pain monster tells you is "You better not go to work today or I'll bite you right in your lower back—and you know what that feels like. Now, drive me home so I can go lay down!" You hear what it says and choose to drive to work anyway, without even bothering to argue or fight with the monster. What do you think happens? Maybe the monster gets mad and starts screaming even louder, saying, "Damn it! I told you not to come here. Do you want me to bite you?" Again, you hear the monster, you listen to what it says, but you choose to go to work anyway. You stop the bus, get out, and spend the day at work. (This is just one example of where you might want to take your bus; alternatively, the destination might involve parenting, homemaking, volunteer work, or anything else that's meaningful to you.)

When you come out, your pain monster is still on the bus and it looks really pissed. You're almost sure it's going to bite you, but you bravely enter the bus anyway. Knowing all the ways your pain monster might try to take revenge on you for not listening to it, you drive your bus home and lie down to go to sleep.

From then on, you do what you want to do instead of what your pain monster tells you to do. You don't ask the monster to leave the bus. You take it right along with you. You just decide that you're going to do what *you* need to do, not in spite of what that pain monster says but with all of its ugly threats and ranting. Like Joe the Bum, you invite your pain monster to stay, but you make it clear that you're going to do whatever you like even with your monster there.

Can you imagine what this might be like? Can you imagine what your pain monster might do in time? What would it be like if you could drive your life bus wherever you wanted to go, harboring pain monsters and old ladies alike? What would that change for you?

WHAT IS COMMITTED ACTION?

In the previous chapter you learned that you could accept difficult aspects of your life in order to make room for yourself to live the way you want to live. You made a conscious choice to accept your pain so that you could start shaping the direction of your life instead of letting your pain be in control of it. You learned that by opening up and embracing that which causes you pain, you can shift the balance from living as your pain dictates to living as *you* wish to. You learned that you could let go of control and holler a mighty *yes!* across the rooftops of the world.

But what is the real value of this? On the one hand, it is nice to be able to find a little wiggle room in your life and loosen the bonds with which your pain has restricted you for so long. But in the end, what does this really give you? Acceptance, like mindfulness, can offer you a change in perspective. It can offer you a new way to look at your experience with pain and your experience as a human being. But independently it doesn't give you the tools you need to enact your valued life every day. You need commitment to achieve that.

It is when you marry acceptance with commitment that you find real power. Acceptance gives you the opportunity to have that realization, as in the example above, where you see that you are in control of your life bus. And that is a powerful and important realization. However, it doesn't take you anywhere unless you make the choice to go somewhere. You have to commit to acting on your own behalf. That means deciding what you want to do and then making a plan to do it. That's what committed action is: choosing to do something and then doing it.

When combined with acceptance, committed action is quite different from the "I'm going to do this no matter what comes up and just grin and bear it" kind of thinking that we've all experimented with. It isn't about keeping your nose to the grindstone or just pushing on in spite of whatever pain you feel. Committed action when married with acceptance gives you the choice to get on your life bus and drive it wherever you want to go, no matter which passengers come on (Hayes, Strosahl, and Wilson 1999).

If you've ever been on a real bus, you know that bus drivers don't go where their passengers tell them. Most of them drive their route no matter who gets on the bus. Sometimes scary passengers get on; sometimes friendly passengers get on. This doesn't have much effect on the driver, who carries any and all passengers along the intended route.

Now it's your turn to do the same thing in regard to your life. It's time for you to take back the steering wheel of your life bus and drive in the direction you want to go. The question is, Where do you want to go?

YOUR VALUES COMPASS POINTS THE WAY

You actually already know where you want to go, and you know exactly what you want to do. You've known these things for some time now. In chapter 3, we explored what sort of life is meaningful to you and helped you build a values compass. We did this early in the book to give you a sense of the possibilities this program offers you. Now that you've developed your defusion, mindfulness, and acceptance skills, it's time to move in the direction you set in your values compass. You have the tools to take charge of your life, so let's get on with it.

Using Your Values Compass to Decide Where to Go

Go back to chapter 3 and look over your values compass again. Take some time to contemplate what you wrote there and make sure that what you said about your values in each of the ten realms accurately reflects what you want your life to be about. If it does, then go ahead and write out your valued life directions again in the spaces below one more time so you can easily reference them in this chapter. If anything has changed about your values or your understanding of them as you've worked through this book, make sure the statements below reflect that new understanding.

Intimate relationships: _____

_____

_____

_____

Parenting: _____

_____

_____

_____

Family relationships: _____

_____

_____

_____

Social relationships: _____

_____

_____

_____

Work: _____

_____

_____

_____

Leisure: _____

_____

_____

_____

Citizenship: _____

_____

_____

_____

Personal growth: _____

_____

_____

_____

Health: _____

_____

_____

_____

Spirituality: _____

_____

_____

_____

Now take a look at your assessment of your values illness, which you determined when you completed your values compass in chapter 3. (The discrepancy between your intentions and your actions in regard to your values is the measure of your values illness.) Are there areas where you feel that you're not truly living your life the way you want to right now? If so, take some notes on that in the space above as well. And again, if anything has changed in this regard since you started working through this book, make sure what you write reflects how you now feel. Above all, just be honest about where you are and how you feel. That way you can make honest and realistic choices about where you want to go.

Now decide on one value that you'd like to work with for the rest of this chapter. The actions you take in regard to that value will be a model for choices you can make in other areas of your life. The rest of this chapter will guide you through a process in regard to that value that will be a template for curing your values illness in other realms. Once you know how to take committed actions in the direction indicated by that value, you can use the same process to lay out a map of all the committed actions you'd like to take in each valued area of your life. To be clear, we're not asking you to choose one and abandon the rest. In fact, we strongly encourage you *not* to do that. Finding a way to move forward in each of your valued directions is important and eventually you'll want to take committed actions in the direction indicated by each of your values.

However, for now start with just one. This may be an area where you suffer from a great deal of values illness or it may not. Either is fine, and what you choose doesn't really matter for the purposes of this chapter. If you feel confident and want to take a big step, choose an aspect of your life that needs a lot of work. Think about doing something in that area that would make you feel vital and alive again. This may provide strong motivation. If you still feel a little bit of trepidation, then work on an area where your values illness is only minor and build up to more challenging areas over time.

Once you've chosen the value you're going to work on in this chapter, write it down in the space below:

_____

_____

Now think about that value and try to come up with a concrete action that would take you one step in that direction. What could you do right now, today, that would allow you to manifest that value in some way? Choose a concrete, achievable goal that would make you feel vital and alive. For example, let's say you want to improve your health by exercising more. You used to love to go to the gym to work out, but since the pain started you just haven't been able to manage it. In this case, it probably isn't realistic to start back on your old routine right away. You need to build back up to where you were before. You need to take gradual steps toward achieving your fitness goals and furthering you along your path toward better health and a happier life. So the single practical step you can take today may be going to the gym and walking on the treadmill for ten minutes. Don't bite off more than you can chew, which is usually counterproductive, but do try to take bold steps in the direction you want to go.

So think in terms of practical steps that will move you down the road toward your value, and when you've decided on the action you're committed to, write it down in the space below:

_____

_____

Congratulations! Just choosing the first action you'll commit to is actually your first step toward the life you value. Now it's time to take the next step.

Just Do It

This next step is fairly easy, but it can be a little intimidating. Whatever action you chose, just go out and do it.

That's it.

There is no magic secret about it. Just go do it now. Don't hesitate.

This is where a lot of people run into trouble. It's all fine and well to theorize about the life you want to live, but actually living it can be a completely different story.

You have the power to choose to act right now, in this very moment, if you wish. There is no one and nothing to stop you from doing this. The distance between writing down what you intend to do in this book and actually doing it is only a hair's breadth. All you have to do is make the commitment to doing whatever it is you've decided to do. You just have to choose to do it, then it's yours. It really *is* that simple.

But this is the point where your mind starts getting loud a lot of the time and telling you what it thinks you need to be doing. As a result, this is where people tend to get stuck. They think about a good committed action they can take in the direction of their values and know it's something they really want to do, but they don't do it because the mind machine starts giving them all sorts of reasons not to. They fall into their content. They start listening to the monsters on the bus (Hayes, Strosahl, and Wilson 1999). They forsake the perspective of the chessboard and start fighting among the chess pieces.

In chapter 8 we'll help you develop strategies and skills for overcoming barriers that may come up for you as you proceed down your valued path. In the meanwhile, there is an important point we need to go ahead and mention in this regard.

This moment, the moment when you take action on your chosen goal, is what you've been working toward in every chapter up to this point in this book. All of the defusion techniques, mindfulness skills, and acceptance strategies are designed so that you can use them in real time. When you make the choice to move in a direction you value, especially if it's a direction you haven't moved in for a long time, there's no question that your mind will start giving you reasons not to do so. It might tell you that you'll end up in pain, that you'll be disappointed, that you'll be unhappy, and so on. Your mind is never going to stop with that blather; that's what it's built to do—it's built to produce content. There can even be some value in that, but it doesn't need to define you and you already know this.

So when you hit places where you feel something inside holding you back from the action you've chosen to take, take a step back and look at that obstacle for what it is, not what it says it is. See if you can breathe it in and embrace it. Then see if you can move in your valued direction, bringing along whatever pain or fear you may have. As long as you choose goals that make you feel truly vital and alive, you'll find that the more times you choose to move in a valued direction with your pain and all that comes with it, the easier it becomes to keep doing so. Behavioral reinforcement is a powerful influence in the lives of human beings.

Remember our discussion of experiential avoidance and how detrimental it is? One of the reasons experiential avoidance has such a profound effect is because it can lead to positive short-term outcomes. When you avoid things and hold your pain at bay, you get some gratification for doing so. You feel relieved because you didn't have to do whatever you avoided. This can lead you to try to escape again and again. Over time, this turns into a vicious cycle and you end up avoiding things even when doing so no longer provides the short-term reward you once gained from it.

Moving in the opposite direction changes this dynamic and creates a positive cycle. Every time you consciously make a committed step in the direction of your values, you derive a sense of true gratification. That doesn't necessarily mean that your choices will always lead to immediate happiness. But if you're mindful of your feelings, if you learn to make choices that make you feel vital and alive, and if you don't do things just because you think you're supposed to, then the committed actions you take will provide positive reinforcement. And each time you do this, choosing to act will get easier and easier.

Throughout your day-to-day life, you act in ways that make you feel vital and alive and you act in ways that don't. To reinforce your committed actions over time, try to make more and more choices that fill you up and make you feel alive. That means you need to start taking more and more steps in the directions you value. So make sure you check in from time to time to see whether the actions you're choosing make you feel vital and alive. Here's an exercise that will help you with this.

EXERCISE: TESTING FOR VITALITY

Over the course of the next few days, try to be mindful of your day-to-day actions and see if you can find out what they are in service of. Try to evaluate whether the choices you make in your day-to-day life make you feel vital and alive. After all, your day-to-day choices and actions are what dictate whether you're leading a life you value or not.

As you enter into an everyday activity, take a moment to evaluate whether you're doing this activity in the service of reducing your pain or to support living your valued life. In the chart below, nonvital means the activity is done for pain relief and vital means that doing the activity supports living your values.

When you've evaluated the activity, make some notes in the worksheet below. Write down the action you took and place a checkmark in the appropriate column depending on whether the activity was vital or nonvital.

Action	Nonvital	Vital

What did you learn from your evaluations? Can you extrapolate to get a sense of what percentage of your daily activities could be deemed vital? If most of the activities you do are, in fact, in the nonvital category, you need to take some committed actions so that you can revitalize your life.

How did you know which activities were vital and which were nonvital? Describe your feelings about each type of activity below.

A vital activity felt _____

_____

_____

_____

A nonvital activity felt _____

_____

_____

_____

Most people say that when they feel vital, they feel as if they are completely alive, vibrating with energy in body, mind, and spirit. When you make decisions about committed actions you wish to take, this sense of vitality should be your guide. In some cases, it may be scary, tickling, and maybe even painful to stand your ground and act on your commitment while your own mind and perhaps even the people around you advise you differently. But remember, it's your life that's at stake here. Would you sacrifice your quality of life and your values because your mind or the people around you disagree with your chosen path?

Keep in mind that the vitality and the energy you receive when you take steps that serve your values are what will reinforce your commitments and make them strong. When you realize you're doing things that make you feel vital and alive, and when you begin to feel the benefits of doing so, it's so much easier to follow through on your commitments. When you realize that you can take these steps while also bringing your chronic pain and everything that comes with it along for the ride, then you're truly in a position to live the life you want to live, no matter what cards you are dealt.

Have you gone ahead and done whatever it was you decided to do earlier in the chapter? If not, go ahead and do so now to test how vital it makes you feel. If you have done it, think about how it felt to take that step. Did it make you feel alive? Imagine that you could feel that alive every day. Imagine what it would be like to get closer and closer to feeling that alive every minute. Wouldn't that be how you want to live? Wouldn't that be a life you could look back on in your final days and think, "That was a life worth living." You can live that life, and you can start today.

LIVING IN THE BULL'S-EYE: TAKING COMMITTED ACTIONS EVERY DAY

Thus far, we've asked you to take one committed step in the direction of the life you value. The next thing to do is to take another step, and then another step, and then another . . . This is how you live your life: step-by-step. Together, those steps delineate your journey and determine where you're headed. So what do you want your life to be about?

Living a valued life isn't a goal. It isn't a destination that you get to and then end the journey. It isn't a game to be won. It's a process—an ongoing process that you live every day for the rest of your life. Notice that you developed a values compass in chapter 3—not a values map, a values board game, or a values maze, but a values compass. A compass doesn't indicate where you are, nor does it indicate your destination. A compass simply keeps you oriented and allows you to be clear about what direction you're headed in. When you use a compass, you look at it to help you choose the direction you'll travel in; it can't guide you to your destination.

That's precisely why we use the values compass metaphor in this book. Values aren't a destination, they're a direction. And you can choose to either move in the direction of your values or not every day you're alive.

The ultimate goal of this chapter, and of this entire book, is to help you start choosing a life you value. We want to give you a way to live in accord with your values every day of your life from here on out. That means committing to a series of actions that will take you in your valued direction; assessing whether or not those actions make you feel vitally alive; changing your course when you need to; and then taking more committed actions. We've developed the following exercise to help you do this.

EXERCISE: THE BULL'S-EYE

This exercise is essentially a committed action worksheet. Over the course of the next week, start living your valued life by taking committed actions and recording your progress on this worksheet. Make a commitment to yourself right now that you'll make at least one committed step in the direction of your values every day for the next week. You'll need seven photocopies of this worksheet for the week. These will be your bull's-eye diary, in which you'll keep track of the committed actions you are taking, assess how vital those actions make you feel, and then refine your next committed action by taking into account what you could do differently that would make you feel more vitally alive.

In this exercise, the bull's-eye represents feeling completely and vitally alive as you take your committed step or as a result of taking that step. Therefore, your goal is to get closer and closer to the bull's-eye—to get closer to living in that space where you feel as vital as you possibly can every single day.

Choose one of the ten life domains we explored in chapter 3 to concentrate on. (It may be easiest to start with the value you chose earlier in the chapter, but if you'd rather focus on something else, that's okay too.) What area would you like to focus on?

_____

_____

Now consider how you could most completely express your values in this area. Write what you envision in the space below. Take into consideration whatever you wrote down earlier in this chapter and in chapter 3 about your values in this domain.

_____

_____

Now come up with an action you could take that would move you one step in your valued direction. (Although you've done this once before, it's time to do it again.)

_____

_____

Now close this book and go out and take the step that you've committed to. Come back to this book when you're done so you can evaluate your action using the bull's-eye below.

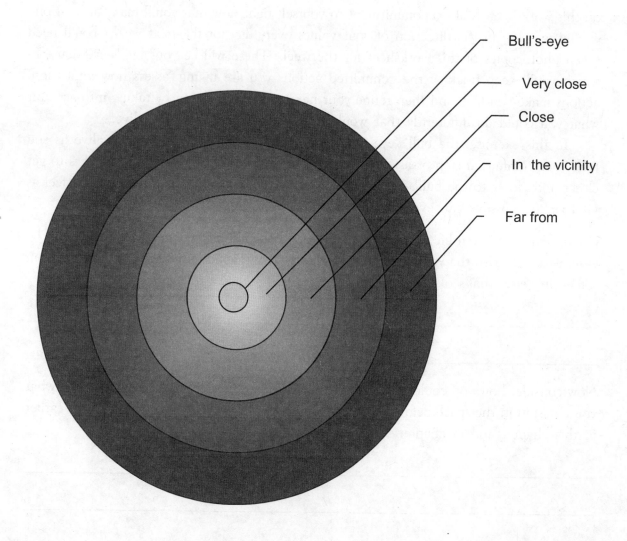

Bull's-eye

Very close

Close

In the vicinity

Far from

Great work! Now it's time to evaluate the step you took. On the dartboard above, there are five levels at which you can rate your action: "far away," "in the vicinity," "close," "very close," and "bull's-eye." Evaluate how your action made you feel and mark an X in the area that most closely represents how close the action brought you to feeling vitally alive.

For example, if you decided to take an action that you thought would move you in the direction of the value you chose, but you didn't feel empowered by the act, you might mark "far away." This is nothing to be ashamed of. It's important information that you'll use below, in the final step of this exercise.

For each committed action you take in your valued direction, mark the appropriate space on the dartboard. In some cases you may get close to feeling completely empowered; other times you may feel that while your choice seemed as though it would move you in your valued direction, it didn't get you as close as you thought it would. Whatever the case, mark the appropriate region on the dartboard and view this as a positive step toward gaining a greater understanding of how you can manifest the life you desire.

If you committed to and followed through on an action that made you feel vibrantly alive, you have hit the bull's-eye. Mark it down and congratulate yourself; ideally, this is where you'd get to with every action you take every day of your life.

If your committed action didn't hit the bull's-eye, ask yourself these questions:

What was it about this experience that resulted in my not feeling completely vitalized?

_____

_____

_____

What could I do that might make me feel I've gotten closer to my valued path?

_____

_____

_____

What is a specific, concrete action I can take in order to achieve this?

_____

_____

_____

Now go out and do *that* action, then go through this entire process once again.

The goal of the above exercise is to help you refine your awareness of the vitality you feel as well as the choices you make about what committed actions to take so that you can live more and more of your life in the bull's-eye. As always, this isn't a measure to judge yourself against. It's simply information that can help you move in a particular direction—the direction of your values.

Keep in mind that you cannot fail when you move in the direction of your values. The only failure is not moving at all. Each step you take provides you with important information you can use to make better and better choices about what you do with your life.

Before moving on, let's hear what Beth and Eric had to say about the bull's-eye exercise.

Beth: *Most of the choices I've made in my life have been based on what others thought was best. For me, this exercise was a totally new experience. Instead of running around trying to live up to others' expectations, I found guidance within myself, my own values, and my own experience. Although this exercise is simple and doesn't require much thought, it's very powerful. The more you do it and experience that feeling of vitality, that feeling of being in the bull's-eye, the less you want to do things for all of your old reasons. That just feels meaningless. I still have a long way to go, but now I know where I'm going and have some experience and information to draw on to help me figure out how to get there.*

Eric: *The whole idea of using the life compass and the bull's-eye was really supportive and helped me get started. The bull's-eye exercise forced me to take a good hard look at what I was up to. It showed me that most of what I did was about avoiding pain, which really felt meaningless and dead. I felt as though my world was getting smaller and smaller. This exercise helped me understand my values and what it means to step up and do what needs to be done to honor those values. It helped me to get back my integrity. I used the bull's-eye and my life compass for a week and then these techniques were in my head. It was easy after that to feel the vitality of making choices that support my values. I sometimes go back to both the compass and the bull's-eye when I feel I'm regressing into old patterns. Although I still have pain, it no longer directs my life—I do.*

BUILDING A TEAM TO SUPPORT YOUR COMMITMENTS

As you change your actions, your behavior, and the course of your life, which you will when taking steps in your valued directions, getting the help and support of people around you is important. As you move away from a life based on avoiding your pain and toward a life based on your values, you will change, and others will notice this. Telling them what's going on for you and asking for their support can be a powerful way to reinforce the work you're doing.

In most cases, becoming more vitally alive by moving in the directions you value will be wonderful for the people around you. It will mean that they get to experience a more complete version of who you are, and that's a wonderful thing. But in some cases, and especially in the short run, others may have a hard time accepting your new behavior. For example, if your priority has been taking care of other people and now you start to take care of yourself a bit more, the people you've been taking care of might not see this as such a wonderful move. Keep in mind that in the long run, they'll see it's all for the best. But in the short run, your changes may be difficult for the people around you.

In the following exercise, think about how the changes you're making in your life by moving in the direction of your values might influence your family, friends, and coworkers, and anyone else who's important to you. Then see if you can find a way that you can commit to helping those around you understand what you're moving toward.

EXERCISE: BUILDING YOUR SUPPORT TEAM

Who do you think will be affected by the changes you're making in your life right now?

_____

_____

_____

How do you think they'll react?

_____

_____

_____

_____

_____

_____

How could you commit to helping these people understand what you're doing?

_____

_____

_____

_____

_____

Hopefully, the preceding exercise will help you predict, prevent, and cope with some of the difficulties you may encounter in your relationships as you take your committed steps toward your values. You may find it helpful to try to foresee conflicts that might arise and to ease these potential difficulties by telling the people in your life about the changes you'll be making and what values you hope to live out by making these changes. Acknowledging others' potential discomfort may be preferable to leaving them wondering about what's going on with you. Here are some tips on how you might communicate with others about the changes you're making:

- Be clear and honest about your values, what you want to do, and what you're doing now. Refer back to your intentions on your life compass for clarity about this, then take a stand for your values and for yourself.

- Talk about yourself and what you want. For example, you might say: "I'm going to start a course in ceramics, because I want to meet others and do things that are creative. Working with others in creative ways gives my life meaning and energy. I'd like to have your support in doing this. Can you stay home and take care of the kids and the household chores one night a week?"

- Invite others who are important to you to be with you and accompany you down your chosen path. This also allows them to experience your increased vitality, and that will assuredly help them support your changes. For example, you might say, "I'm making a commitment to exercise regularly at the gym; would you like to join me?"

- Be flexible and use the defusion, mindfulness, and acceptance techniques you've learned in this book in the moment when you need to. If people react negatively to your commitments or behavior changes, try to make room for their reactions and simply accept them without backing off from your commitments.

- Honor your values and be persistent in honoring them and searching for the vitality you deserve to experience in this life.

LIVING A LIFE YOU VALUE EVERY DAY

If you've made it to this point in the book, we want to congratulate you. You've done some incredible work! You have now worked through the heart of this program. You know how to use defusion, mindfulness, and acceptance techniques to help you make choices to live a life you value with your pain, instead of living a life designed to avoid your pain. Now that you've learned all of this and begun to put it to work in your day-to-day life, you just need to keep doing it, day in and day out. Living your values means choosing meaningful, vital actions every day. That's the kind of life we want for you, and we hope we've helped you move in that direction.

Before we send you off to pursue your valued life on your own, we want to offer you one more set of techniques that can be helpful. Sometimes when people run into barriers, they stumble and stray from the ACT path. It's helpful to be prepared for that possibility, so in the final chapter we'll teach you what to do when you encounter barriers. (And there are always barriers.)

CHAPTER 8

What's Holding You Back?

Because we are all human, and life being what it is, you will face barriers on the road to your valued life. There's no way around that. You're going to run into situations where life is difficult, where the pain seems overwhelming, and where you start to fall back into your mental content. Sometimes you will stray from the path of mindfulness and acceptance, and sometimes you'll take steps that don't lead you in your valued direction. Sometimes you might not take any steps at all. The question is, What are you going to do in those situations?

The short answer to this question is that you are going to employ all the same techniques you've learned about throughout the course this book. At this point, you actually already know what to do when barriers come up. You've been practicing it and the process is simple: Defuse from your thoughts and see them for what they are, not what they say they are. Take the observer perspective and look at the situation from the eyes of that most basic and essential part of yourself. Open up and embrace the barrier that obstructs your path. Then reflect on your values and commit to taking steps in the direction of your values, bringing your pain, mental chatter, and other barriers along with you. In essence, the way to overcome barriers is to do exactly what you have already been doing.

However, because barriers are inevitable, it can be helpful to consider in advance what barriers you think you might face and come up with ways you may handle those barriers. In this chapter, we'll help you develop an action plan you can take when you face barriers on your path to a valued life, or when you stray from the ACT mind-set and skills.

OBSTACLES IN A RIVER

Have you ever floated down a river in an inner tube? If you have, you know that all sorts of surprises come up as you float down the river, some nice and some not so nice. There are areas where you can just lie back in pure bliss and enjoy the water and sunshine. But there are also dangerous areas: swift currents, tumultuous rapids, fallen logs, and big underwater rocks that you can't always see from the surface. One thing is certain: You can't control these challenging parts of the river, and you may not even be able to predict them. A great many of these obstacles are, in fact, under the water, and you cannot see or influence them. Rocks and downed trees can turn up where you least expect them. If you worry about the dangers all the time, you won't fully enjoy the benign parts of the river float. The key is to be mindfully present as you float down the river, making the most of the quiet stretches and remaining alert during the challenging sections, while also appreciating the rewards the difficult sections offer. It's the same in life: It's important to partake fully of the joys of life and to deal with the challenges, barriers, and dangers as they arise.

How do you approach the dangers? Most people's natural reaction to the dangerous parts of the river is to try to gain control by putting their feet down on the river bottom. If you've done this, you know that putting your feet down can be extremely dangerous. Your feet can get caught among rocks while the rapids carry the rest of you away. You get bruised, broken, or worse, and the rest of the ride is ruined.

Your best bet is to relax, allow the current to carry you along, and deal with dangerous spots as they show up. Sticking your feet down to the bottom to gain control because you're afraid of what might happen is likely to get you into far greater trouble. This is a good illustration of why your mind is not always your best advisor. Your minds screams at you to put your feet down and get control but it's actually in your best interests to override that warning. In order for you to have the best experience, you need to let go of those reflexes to control.

As with anything, experience in floating down a river in an inner tube teaches you certain things. Eventually you learn how to let go of control a little bit and let the river take you where it wants to go. You learn to keep your feet up and not try to interrupt your progress even if you aren't going exactly where you thought you'd go. You learn to go with the flow and deal with problems as they arise.

If you float down the same river a number of times, you start to know where the trouble spots are. In time you can predict places where you'll face rough water. And as you now know, those are precisely the times when you need to open up and accept wherever the water takes you, rather than trying to control the river.

EXERCISE: IDENTIFYING YOUR OBSTACLES

Take a moment to imagine you're in an inner tube right now, floating down the river of your life. You've chosen the river you want to be on, and you're floating in the direction of your values. The ride is peaceful and beautiful for the most part, but you know there are places where it's going to get rough.

As you imagine floating down this river of your life, making committed choices to move in the directions you value, what obstacles pop up in your head to stop you? Are there thoughts that intrude on your commitment to your values right now? Do you predict future encounters and events that you fear will be difficult? You've been on this river before. Think about places where you've encountered problems in the past. Where are some of the obstacles you expect to encounter on your path to a valued life? (An example from Beth follows if you need help getting going.)

Obstacle 1: _____

_____

Obstacle 2: _____

_____

Obstacle 3: _____

_____

Obstacle 4: _____

_____

Obstacle 5: _____

_____

Obstacle 6: _____

_____

Obstacle 7: _____

_____

Obstacle 8: _____

_____

BETH'S OBSTACLES

Obstacle 1: *You failed in school before and you have trouble remembering names and phone numbers now. How are you ever going to make it through college?*

Obstacle 2: *You're over-the-hill and you'll look stupid among those young college kids. Stay home, where you belong.*

Obstacle 3: *Your family needs a new car and a new washing machine, plus you have to save for the kids' college education. Why should you spend money on you, especially now?*

Obstacle 4: *If you have any time left over, you should be taking care of your poor mother-in-law instead of thinking about yourself. She really has problems.*

Obstacle 5: *The kids are at a very sensitive age and they need their mom at home. If you really need to go back to school, you can wait until they go off to college. Their needs come first.*

Obstacle 6: *Your husband is feeling very stressed-out at work and needs your support. If you go back to school, you'll stress him even more. He's the main breadwinner and you need to be there for him.*

Obstacle 7: *You know that you can't sit through lectures. What are you going to do, stand up? If you take painkillers, you won't remember a thing, so you know you can't do that.*

Obstacle 8: *You have never been especially smart and never got great grades in school. What makes you think you can even pass these college courses? Give up now before you embarrass yourself.*

EXERCISE: IDENTIFYING OLD COPING STRATEGIES

Look back at the obstacles you listed above. If you've encountered any of these in the past, think back and remember some of the ways you dealt with those obstacles before. If one of your obstacles is your pain, consider all of the ways you've tried to cope with or fight your pain in the past. Use the spaces below to write about how you've coped with each obstacle in the past. If any of the obstacles you listed aren't things you've encountered in the past, then you need not complete this part of the exercise for those particular obstacles.

Old coping strategies for obstacle 1: _____

_____

Old coping strategies for obstacle 2: _____

_____

Old coping strategies for obstacle 3: _____

_____

Old coping strategies for obstacle 4: _____

_____

Old coping strategies for obstacle 5: _____

_____

Old coping strategies for obstacle 6: _____

_____

Old coping strategies for obstacle 7: _____

_____

Old coping strategies for obstacle 8: _____

_____

EXERCISE: BETH'S OLD COPING STRATEGIES

Old coping strategies for obstacle 1 (previous failure in school): *Laugh it off, stress out, or discipline myself very harshly.*

Old coping strategies for obstacle 2 (over-the-hill): *Buy cosmetics and try to look younger. Go on diets and try to lose weight.*

Old coping strategies for obstacle 3 (financial problems): *Get a part-time job working the night shift. Take in neighbors' kids after school for money.*

Old coping strategies for obstacle 4 (mother-in-law's needs): *Sleep less. Change the times I wake up and go to bed to make more time to help my mother-in-law.*

Old coping strategies for obstacle 5 (kids' needs): *Don't pursue my own growth; just be there for the kids.*

Old coping strategies for obstacle 6 (husband's needs): *Wait until his situation is more stable, then think about my education.*

Old coping strategies for obstacle 7 (pain): *Start with a shorter evening course that doesn't require sitting so long.*

Old coping strategies for obstacle 8 (not smart enough): *Start at a lower level, maybe at a high school level, where I don't risk failing. That will help me see if I can do it.*

EXERCISE: DEVELOPING COMMITTED
ACTION PLANS FOR OBSTACLES

Now go back and review the list you made above of some of the obstacles you think you might face in the river of your life. Using the information and techniques in this book, can you see ways that you might be able to be more mindful and accept these obstacles as a natural part of your valued life? Do you think you can accept this obstacle, carry it with you, and still act in ways that support your values? Think in specifics. Are there particular techniques in this book that you've found useful for embracing your pain and taking it with you as you journey in the direction of a valued life? Though pain may be one of your biggest obstacles, it is just one among many you'll face in this lifetime. The techniques that work well for you for accepting and embracing pain should work well for other obstacles, too.

In the space below, develop an action plan for each obstacle you listed above. Think of ways that you can let go of control, flow with the river, defuse from your thoughts, be more mindful, accept the obstacles in your path, and continue to move in your valued directions. (Again, an example from Beth follows.)

Acceptance and committed action plan for obstacle 1: _____

_____

_____

_____

Acceptance and committed action plan for obstacle 2: _____

_____

_____

_____

Acceptance and committed action plan for obstacle 3: _____

_____

_____

_____

Acceptance and committed action plan for obstacle 4: _____

_____

_____

_____

Acceptance and committed action plan for obstacle 5: _____

_____

_____

_____

Acceptance and committed action plan for obstacle 6: _____

_____

_____

_____

Acceptance and committed action plan for obstacle 7: _____

_____

_____

_____

Acceptance and committed action plan for obstacle 8: _____

_____

_____

_____

Remember to come back to these action plans when you actually do face these obstacles in the river of your life. They are here for you to use so that you can continue floating peacefully down the river.

EXERCISE: BETH'S COMMITTED ACTION PLANS FOR HER OBSTACLES

Acceptance and committed action plan for obstacle 1 (previous failure in school): I *appreciate the reminders of my previous negative experience from school. I understand that you are trying to protect me from that happening again. Thank you. I'm going to keep those thoughts next to me as I go forward into the scary realm of educational challenges and trust that I'll solve the problems that come up rather than not give myself this chance. It's better that I try and fail than shut off this possibility. I'll start filling out school applications on Monday and open this door for myself.*

Acceptance and committed action plan for obstacle 2 (over-the-hill): I *understand that you're reminding me of my age and the age difference between me and my classmates because you don't want me to make a fool of myself. I do look older and act differently, and at the same time I believe my classmates and I can enrich each other from our different life perspectives. I commit to bringing up these differences at our first meeting and telling them how I feel about it.*

Acceptance and committed action plan for obstacle 3 (financial problems): I *understand that you don't want us to be poor or get into financial difficulties as has happened in the past. It's very scary to be poor and not know how you'll pay the bills. I've learned how to prioritize and make ends meet over the years, and I feel confident that I can set up a budget for the three years it will take me to get my degree so that our family won't suffer economically. I commit to taking responsibility for setting up a three-year budget for our family.*

Acceptance and committed action plan for obstacle 4 (mother-in-law's needs): My *mother-in-law does need help, and I commit to looking for a service that offers just the type of help she needs. I'll put aside time for me to be with her and show her that I love her and want to be with her. Someone else can see to her daily needs.*

Acceptance and committed action plan for obstacle 5 (kids' needs): Being *present for my children is one of my most deeply felt values and I appreciate your reminding me about what is important. With that in mind, I commit to considering all my activities at home and prioritizing time with my children. I can be sensitive to their needs and have time for them and still make time to go to school. This will probably mean that the whole family will have to take more responsibility for daily household chores.*

Acceptance and committed action plan for obstacle 6 (husband's needs): I *value supporting Bill in any difficulties that he has. Thanks for reminding me never to be so caught up in my own life that I forget and take for granted the value of our marriage and the importance of Bill's health and welfare. I see my going back to school as a way to ease the strain and responsibility of his being the main breadwinner. I commit to making up a renewed marriage contract where I specify my long-term goals and describe how taking this step will contribute to vitalizing our marriage and reaffirming our love for each other.*

Acceptance and committed action plan for obstacle 7 (pain): *I admit that sitting has been a problem and there is a lot of sitting in school, so I appreciate your warning me about that. I commit to going to a physical therapist and telling her just what I need to be able to do and for how long in order to get my degree. I'll do whatever exercises I need to do or use the aids I need to use.*

Acceptance and committed action plan for obstacle 8 (not smart enough): *I appreciate your wanting to protect me from looking less smart than others. I may, in fact, have more trouble learning than my classmates, and I am rusty from not going to school for such a long time. If I keep that thought close to me, I'll be alert to this difficulty and can ask for help when I need it. I commit to being mindful of any difficulties I may run into and asking for help as soon as that happens rather than ignoring the situation or criticizing or punishing myself.*

BACK ON THE BUS

In chapter 7, we introduced you to the bus metaphor (Hayes, Strosahl, and Wilson 1999). In it we propositioned what it might be like to be the driver on your life bus—a bus where, unfortunately but inevitably, monsters and other ghoulish passengers are getting on and off at their whim. In this chapter, we'll expand the metaphor to help you develop more action plans to help you with your barriers.

EXERCISE: DEVELOPING ACT STRATEGIES FOR DEALING WITH UNRULY PASSENGERS ON YOUR LIFE BUS

Imagine you're back on your bus and you're getting ready to go out for a drive. It's a beautiful day, and you decide you want to drive down a road you haven't been on in a while. You want to drive in the direction of your values.

The first thing you have to decide is which value you want to move toward. Go back to your values compass in chapter 3 and the work you did on committed action in chapter 7 and choose the direction you want to move in. Remember, this is what the sign on the front of your bus is going to say, and everyone and everything that gets on your bus is going to have to move in that direction with you.

When you've decided on your valued direction, write it in the space below:

_____

_____

Now that you've decided on your direction, you need a route to follow. Choose a few committed action steps; these will be the stops on the bus route you're designing. Think in terms of actions that will take you in the direction of the value you stated above, and describe what you intend to do in the spaces below. If you need some help with this part of the exercise, take a look at the example from Beth, below, or review chapter 7.

Committed action 1: _____

_____

_____

_____

Committed action 2: _____

_____

_____

Committed action 3: _____

_____

_____

_____

Committed action 4: _____

_____

_____

_____

Now that you've established your route, you can get on the road. Take a moment to imagine that you're on your bus and that you're driving in the direction of the action you want to take. Up ahead is your first stop, the first committed action you listed above. You pull over and stop the bus, and right when you stop a monster jumps in, sits right next to you, and starts screaming at you. It's telling you all the reasons you won't be able to take your first committed action. Take a few minutes to listen to this monster and hear what it's saying. In the space below, write down what the monster is telling you.

Monster 1 yells: _____

_____

_____

_____

Now take a few minutes to think about ways that you might handle this monster. You could decide to fight with it, but you know that isn't going to get you anywhere. You'll just end up spending all your time fighting with this monster rather than taking committed actions or driving in your valued directions. You could do what the monster tells you to do, but that would mean changing your course and not taking the action you committed to.

Try to think about some ways that you could accept what this monster is yelling at you and still engage in the action you've committed to. Try to use exercises from this book to develop specific responses to the barriers you foresee. If you have trouble with this part of the exercise, take a look at the example from Beth, below.

Acceptance and commitment strategy for monster 1: _____

_____

_____

_____

Good. Now imagine the same thing happens at each stop on the route you've plotted. Every time you pull over to take a valued action, another monster gets on and starts yelling at you. How do you handle each of these situations?

Monster 2 yells: _____

_____

_____

_____

Acceptance and commitment strategy for monster 2: _____

_____

_____

_____

Monster 3 yells: _____

_____

_____

_____

Acceptance and commitment strategy for monster 3: _____

_____

_____

_____

Monster 4 yells: _____

_____

_____

_____

Acceptance and commitment strategy for monster 4: _____

_____

_____

_____

BETH'S ACT STRATEGIES FOR DEALING WITH UNRULY PASSENGERS ON HER LIFE BUS

It might be helpful or interesting for you to see how Beth completed the same exercise when she was in ACT therapy for her chronic pain problem. Here are Beth's committed actions, what she heard the monsters yelling at her, and how she chose to deal with what they said.

Committed action 1: *Call the admissions office and make an appointment to see what I need to do to finish my degree.*

Committed action 2: *Tell my family that I want to go back to school and make a plan for what needs to change at home, like a new distribution of household chores to facilitate this change.*

Committed action 3: *Go to my physical therapist, tell her my plan, and see if she can help me figure out what exercises I can do to help me sit through those long hours in class.*

Committed action 4: *Work with a financial advisor to plan a three-year family budget that includes me going back to school and then present it to the family.*

Committed action 5: *Check the course requirements for my degree to see if any are similar to courses I've had trouble with in the past. If so, I'll make an appointment with the guidance counselor right away about getting any extra tutoring I might need.*

Monster 1 yells: *Are you kidding? You're way too old. It's too late for you.*

Acceptance and commitment strategy for monster 1: *I'll use the exercise on the arrogance of words. I'll say "old" one hundred times and see what happens to it then. I'll get into the perspective of the observer self and turn up my acceptance dial. Then I'll take this idea that I'm too old with me in the direction of my values.*

Monster 2 yells: *Think of your kids! Your kids will suffer. Wait until they've grown up, then you can think of yourself.*

Acceptance and commitment strategy for monster 2: *In my heart I know my kids love me. I can tell myself, "This is me thinking my kids will suffer." Then I can accept that thought as a thought, not as a real statement, and move toward my valued life.*

Monster 3 yells: *Taking care of your pain is a full-time job. Get rid of the pain first before you even think of doing anything else.*

Acceptance and commitment strategy for monster 3: *I've faced a lot of pain in my seated mindfulness exercises. It might not be as much as the pain I feel at other times, but my practice has taught me I can be mindful of the pain and accept it rather than fight against it. I know there's a part of me that's always safe and will always be with me no matter how much pain I have. I'll look at my pain from this perspective and see myself as the chessboard and the pain as simply a piece on the board. Then I'll make decisions that I want to make, not decisions that this pain monster tells me to make.*

Monster 4 yells: *You can't afford to get an education; you can hardly get by now. How will that work? This would be a really poor investment.*

Acceptance and commitment strategy for monster 4: *The idea that I don't have enough money is just a thought. I am competent and I know there are ways I can make money to pay for school. I can take this thought that I don't have enough money with me as just a thought and go to school with it.*

Monster 5 yells: *Don't you remember the time you failed that math test in the ninth grade? You're not smart enough to get an education. You'll make a fool of yourself among all those sharp young minds.*

Acceptance and commitment strategy for monster 5: *"Failure" is a big word. But it's still just a word. If it had a shape and size, it would be a huge wall. If it had a color, it would be black. It smells of horse shit and has a deep and terrible voice. It makes me afraid, but I can make room for this fear in myself. I can give it a home and carry it with me toward the life that I value.*

ACCEPT, COMMIT, TAKE ACTION

And now we close as we opened. Though we've covered a lot of ground, given you many exercises, and helped you develop some new skills, in the end this book is about three basic and interrelated concepts you can use to live a life beyond pain: acceptance, commitment, and taking action. By now you should have a good understanding of how those three concepts work together to form a powerful strategy. You can use this strategy, along with the other tools and skills we've helped you develop, to face the barriers in your life from an open and compassionate stance. This will allow you to move in the directions that you most cherish in life. When you face the inevitable obstacles that the river of your life presents, remember to accept by opening your mind and your heart to the truth of who you are and what you value. Commit to leading the life that you most want to lead, and take committed action in your valued directions. If you do this, you'll live a truly full life, one where your pain is but a small piece of the complex and expansive totality of your being.

CONCLUSION

Living Beyond Your Pain

A path lies open before you now, and the choices you make are your own. We can't tell you what decisions to make, and what you end up doing on this road doesn't have anything to do with us. You are on your own to live your life as you will. We've helped you as far down the path as we can in this book. Now it's time for you to walk away and live out your values every day.

We hope we've helped you to open up a life that had become closed; to vitalize a life that was withering; to realize that you are not your pain and that you can be whatever you choose to be. Living the life you value isn't some gift that comes from the sky and it doesn't involve some mystical moment of insight. It's about the choices you make every day and the actions you take that reflect those choices. Life doesn't just happen. We make it happen, and we can move in the directions we wish if we choose to act in accord with our values.

Letting go of the rope in your tug-of-war with pain can be an incredibly liberating experience, freeing you to do exactly what you want to do. When you use the tools we've given you for living beyond your pain, nothing has to be a barrier; everything you experience can help inform your journey on your path to a valued life.

Every day offers new challenges. And every day your path opens up before you with more richness, complexity, and rewards. It doesn't end until you end. The you that is you and has always been you is truly boundless.

In his 1994 inaugural speech, Nelson Mandela quoted Marianne Williamson on the human condition:

> Our deepest fear is not that we are inadequate. Our deepest fear is that we are powerful beyond measure. It is our light, not our darkness, that most frightens us. We ask ourselves, "Who am I to be brilliant, gorgeous, talented, fabulous?" Actually, who are you *not* to be? You are a child of God. Your playing small does not serve the world. There is nothing enlightened about shrinking so that other people won't feel insecure around you. We are born to make manifest the glory of God that is within us. It is not just in some of us, it is in everyone. And as we let our light shine, we give others the permission to do the same. As we are liberated from our fears, our presence liberates others.

There is no end to what you might do and the roads you might take. Pain need not be a barrier. Open up and let your light shine.

References

Andersson, G. 1997. The epidemiology of spinal disorders. In *The Adult Spine: Principles and Practice*, 2nd edition, ed. J. Frymoyer, pp. 93-141. New York: Raven Press.

Arbus, L., B. Fajadet, D. Aubert, M. Moore, and E. Goldberger. 1990. Activity of tetrazepam (Myolastan) in low back pain: A double-blind trial vs. placebo. *Clinical Trials Journal* 27:258-267.

Asfour, S., T. Khlil, S. Waly, M. Goldberg, R. Rosomoff, and H. Rosomoff. 1990. Biofeedback in back muscle strengthening. *Spine* 15:510-513.

Bigos, S., O. Bowyer, A. Braen, K. Brown, R. Deyo, S. Haldeman, et al. 1994. Acute low back problems in adults. *Clinical Practice Guidelines* 14 (AHCPR Publication No. 95-0642). Rockville, MD: U.S. Agency for Health Care Policy and Research.

Brattberg, G. 1993. Back pain and headache in Swedish schoolchildren: A longitudinal study. *Pain Clinic* 6:157-162.

Brattberg, G. 1994. The incidence of back pain and headache among Swedish school-children. *Quality of Life Research* 67:29-34.

Dahl, J., K. G. Wilson, and A. Nilsson. 2004. Acceptance and Commitment Therapy and the treatment of persons at risk for long-term disability resulting from stress and pain symptoms: A preliminary randomized trial. *Behavior Therapy* 35:785-802.

Davis, M., E. R. Eshelman, and M. McKay. 2000. *The Relaxation and Stress Reduction Workbook,* 5th edition. Oakland, CA: New Harbinger Publications.

Donaldson, S., D. Romney, M. Donaldson, and D. Skubick. 1994. Randomized study of the application of single motor unit biofeedback training to chronic low back pain. *Journal of Occupational Rehabilitation* 4:23-37.

Gregg, J. 2004. Development of an acceptance-based treatment for the self-management of diabetes. Unpublished doctoral dissertation, University of Nevada, Reno.

Gutiérrez, O., C. Luciano, M. Rodríguez, and B. C. Fink. 2004. Comparison between an acceptance-based and a cognitive-control-based protocol for coping with pain. *Behavior Therapy* 35:767-784.

Hackett, G., D. Seddon, and D. Kaminski. 1988. Electroacupuncture compared with paracetamol for acute low back pain. *Practitioner* 232:163-164.

Hayes, S. C. 2004. Acceptance and Commitment Therapy, Relational Frame Theory, and the third wave of behavioral and cognitive therapies. *Behavior Therapy* 35:639-665.

Hayes, S. C., and K. D. Strosahl, eds. 2005. *A Practical Guide to Acceptance and Commitment Therapy.* New York: Springer-Verlag.

Hayes, S. C., K. D. Strosahl, and K. G. Wilson. 1999. *Acceptance and Commitment Therapy: An Experiential Approach to Behavior Change.* New York: Guilford Press.

Heffner, M., and G. H. Eifert. 2004. *The Anorexia Workbook: How to Accept Yourself, Heal Suffering, and Reclaim Your Life.* Oakland, CA: New Harbinger Publications.

Herman, E., R. Williams, P. Stratford, A. Fargas-Babjak, and M. Trott. 1994. A randomized controlled trial of TENS (Codetron) to determine its benefits in a rehabilitation program for acute occupational low back pain. *Spine* 19:561-568.

Luciano, C., J. C. Visdómine, O. Gutiérrez, and F. Montesinos. 2001. ACT and chronic pain. *Análisis y Modificación de Conducta* 27:473-502.

Matsumo, S., K. Kaneda, and Y. Nohara. 1991. Clinical evaluation of ketoprofen (Orudis) in lumbago: A double blind comparison with diclofenac sodium. *British Journal of Clinical Practice* 35:266.

McCracken, L. M., and C. Eccleston. 2003. Coping or acceptance: What to do about chronic pain. *Pain* 105:197-204.

Merskey, H., and N. Bogduk, eds. 1994. *Classification of Chronic Pain: Descriptions of Chronic Pain Syndromes and Definitions of Pain Terms.* 2nd edition. Seattle: IASP.

Nachemson, A., and E. Jonsson. 2000. Inledning [Introduction]. In *SBU-rapport, Ont i ryggen, ont i nacken* [Pain in Back, Pain in Neck], vol. 1, pp. 33-43. Stockholm: SBU.

Newton-John, T., S. Spence, and D. Schotte. 1995. Cognitive-behavioral therapy versus EMG biofeedback in the treatment of chronic low back pain. *Behaviour Research and Therapy* 33:691-697.

Postacchini, F., M. Facchini, and P. Palieri. 1988. Efficacy of various forms of conservative treatment in low back pain: A comparative study. *Neuro-Orthopedics* 6:28-35.

Raspe, H. 1993. Back pain. In *Epidemiology of the Rheumatic Diseases*, ed. A. Silman and M. C. Hoch, pp. 330-374. Oxford: Oxford University Press.

Skekelle, P. 1997. The epidemiology of low back pain. In *Clinical Anatomy and Management of Low Back Pain*, ed. L. Giles and K. Singer, pp. 18-31. London: Butterworth Heinemann.

Van Tulder, M., M. Goossens, and A. Nachemson. 2000. Kroniska ländryggsbesvär: Konservativ behandling [Chronic low back pain: Conservative treatment]. In *SBU-rapport, Ont i ryggen, ont i nacken* [Pain in Back, Pain in Neck], vol. 2, pp. 17-113. Stockholm: SBU.

Waddell, G., and A. Norlund. 2000. System för socialförsäkring en internationell jämförelse [System for social health insurance, an international comparison]. In *SBU-rapport, Ont i ryggen, ont i nacken* [Pain in Back, Pain in Neck], vol. 2, pp. 311-389. Stockholm: SBU.

Zettle, R., and S. Hayes. 1986. Dysfunctional control by client verbal behavior: The context of reason giving. *Analysis of Verbal Behavior* 4:30-38.

JoAnne Dahl, Ph.D., is senior lecturer and associate professor of psychology at the University of Uppsala in Uppsala, Sweden. She is a prominent acceptance and commitment therapy (ACT) researcher who specializes in the use of ACT to treat chronic pain and epilepsy. She travels internationally to conduct ACT workshops and training sessions for professionals. She also continues to research the use of ACT to treat chronic pain and other conditions.

Tobias Lundgren, MS, is a licensed clinical psychologist with a specialization in cognitive behavioral therapy. He is active both as a clinician and researcher of behavior medicine. He has carried out applications of ACT in the clinical research areas of epilepsy, diabetes, and chronic pain. Lundgren works out of the Department of Psychology at the University of Uppsala in Uppsala, Sweden, but he has conducted clinical research with epilepsy clinics and organizations in Pune, India, and Johannesburg and Cape Town, South Africa. Besides clinical research, Tobias conducts educational workshops and clinical trainings and supervises staff members of treatment homes.

Some Other
New Harbinger Titles

The Cyclothymia Workbook, Item 383X, $18.95

The Matrix Repatterning Program for Pain Relief, Item 3910, $18.95

Transforming Stress, Item 397X, $10.95

Eating Mindfully, Item 3503, $13.95

Living with RSDS, Item 3554 $16.95

The Ten Hidden Barriers to Weight Loss, Item 3244 $11.95

The Sjogren's Syndrome Survival Guide, Item 3562 $15.95

Stop Feeling Tired, Item 3139 $14.95

Responsible Drinking, Item 2949 $18.95

The Mitral Valve Prolapse/Dysautonomia Survival Guide, Item 3031 $14.95

Stop Worrying Abour Your Health, Item 285X $14.95

The Vulvodynia Survival Guide, Item 2914 $15.95

The Multifidus Back Pain Solution, Item 2787 $12.95

Move Your Body, Tone Your Mood, Item 2752 $17.95

The Chronic Illness Workbook, Item 2647 $16.95

Coping with Crohn's Disease, Item 2655 $15.95

The Woman's Book of Sleep, Item 2493 $14.95

The Trigger Point Therapy Workbook, Item 2507 $19.95

Fibromyalgia and Chronic Myofascial Pain Syndrome, second edition, Item 2388 $19.95

Kill the Craving, Item 237X $18.95

Rosacea, Item 2248 $13.95

Thinking Pregnant, Item 2302 $13.95

Shy Bladder Syndrome, Item 2272 $13.95

Help for Hairpullers, Item 2329 $13.95

Coping with Chronic Fatigue Syndrome, Item 0199 $13.95

The Stop Smoking Workbook, Item 0377 $17.95

Multiple Chemical Sensitivity, Item 173X $16.95

Breaking the Bonds of Irritable Bowel Syndrome, Item 1888 $14.95

Parkinson's Disease and the Art of Moving, Item 1837 $16.95

The Addiction Workbook, Item 0431 $18.95

The Interstitial Cystitis Survival Guide, Item 2108 $15.95

Call **toll free, 1-800-748-6273,** or log on to our online bookstore at **www.newharbinger.com** to order. Have your Visa or Mastercard number ready. Or send a check for the titles you want to New Harbinger Publications, Inc., 5674 Shattuck Ave., Oakland, CA 94609. Include $4.50 for the first book and 75¢ for each additional book, to cover shipping and handling. (California residents please include appropriate sales tax.) Allow two to five weeks for delivery.

Prices subject to change without notice.